Tai Herbalism

T0363807

TAI HERBALISM

Susan Conway

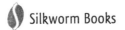 Silkworm Books

ISBN 978-616-215-205-4 (Paperback)

First edition published in 2024 by
Silkworm Books
430/58 M. 7, T. Mae Hia, Chiang Mai 50100, Thailand
info@silkwormbooks.com
www.silkwormbooks.com

Typeset in Minion Pro 11 pt. by Silk Type

Printed and bound in the United States by Lightning Source

Contents

Background vii

Chapter 1: Prescriptions for Making Pills 1

  1. Prescriptions with Ingredients for Making Pills 1

  2. Prescriptions that Include Pills Ground up with Other Ingredients 5

  3. Prescriptions with Ingredients Excluding Pills 8

  4. Controlling Evil Spirits, Ghosts, and Witches 24

Chapter 2: Mystical Diagrams (*Yantra*) 39

  1. Folio 148 41

  2. Folio 149 42

  3. Folio 150 43

  4. Folio 151 45

  5. Folio 152 47

  6. Folio 153 48

  7. Folio 154 49

  8. Folio 155–156 50

  9. Folio 157 52

  10. Folio 163 53

  11. Folio 164 54

  Conclusion 56

Chapter 3: Magic Spells (*Katha*) 61

Glossary 65

Bibliography 69

Medicinal Index 73

Acknowledgments 81

Background

There is a saying among minority people, 'to annihilate my culture and identity you must first destroy my language and writing.'[1] Through intentional political policy or simple ignorance and neglect, minorities all over the world remain at risk of losing or have already lost their languages and unique forms of writing. In the United Kingdom, Welsh language and culture was under threat until constructive measures were adopted to reverse the trend. Today, the Welsh language is thriving. It is taught in schools and many citizens are bilingual. Depriving the rights of people to communicate in their own languages and writing diminishes us all. We are denied an understanding of the past as seen through their eyes, not always interpreted by outsiders. This book highlights a case in point, a manuscript written in a particular form of language and script in danger of extinction with, at most, only a handful of elderly people in Shan State in Myanmar able to read it. But that is not the only reason this manuscript is important. It provides a fascinating insight into Shan herbal medicines and magico-religious belief systems practised in the nineteenth century. It also provides opportunity for comparison. Animals and plants flourished in the forests of nineteenth-century Shan State but in the twenty-first century many are extinct or in danger of extinction. At a practical level, the manuscript gives insight into how the Shan treated physical and mental illness.

---

1. The term 'minority' in this context means a culturally, ethnically, or racially distinct group.

The people who produced this manuscript are Tai who inhabit Shan State, an eastern region of Myanmar, called Burma in the nineteenth century. They are referred to as Shan although many prefer to be called Tai. I use the term Shan to mean Tai of the Shan State. The Tai share a common heritage with other Tai people across Assam, southwest China, Laos, and Thailand. Their fascinating culture is based on a belief system that incorporates Theravada Buddhism, spirit religion, cosmology, astrology, numerology, and the power of nature and sacred objects.[2] Spirit religion involves belief in mystical, supernatural entities. Some are positive and help protect against disease and misfortune. Others are negative spirits that cause misfortune. Positive spirits act as a superior moral force, guiding humans in their relationship with negative spirits. Evil spirits can be wandering ghosts, particularly dangerous when forced from the body of someone who dies in violent circumstances, such as a murder victim, or a woman who dies in childbirth.

This manuscript is part of a collection of Shan artefacts in the Horniman Museum in London. The museum was founded by Frederick Horniman, a British tea trader and avid collector whose mission was to 'illustrate natural history and the arts and handicrafts of various peoples of the world'. The manuscript was collected around 1860 when Horniman travelled in Asia, including to Burma, to add to his collection. Over the years, his collection expanded and became the foundation of the Horniman Museum. We know from the accession number nn12674, 'nn' meaning 'no number', that this manuscript entered the collection in the 1860s.[3]

I discovered the manuscript while working in the Horniman Museum store, searching for relevant material for a book on the culture and history of the Shan people.[4] The manuscript was listed among the museum's index

2. Phrakru Wimonsilapakij of Mahachulalongkornrajavidyalaya University provided this insight into the Tai belief system.

3. Information provided by Dr Fiona Kerlogue, anthropologist, the Horniman Museum, London.

4. Susan Conway, *The Shan: Culture, Arts and Crafts*, Bangkok: River Books, 2006.

cards. This was a time before museum records were accessible online. The index card stated the manuscript was circa nineteenth century and described as a 'Shan Bible'. I assumed from this description that it was a copy of a Christian bible translated by missionaries into Shan language, a common practice when European and American missionaries were proselytising in the region. I doubted it was of interest for my book but added it to the request list to take a quick look.

When the 'Shan Bible' came up from the museum store it turned out to be something quite different, certainly not a Christian bible nor a book in the Western sense. It is a manuscript, made according to local tradition from the shredded and pulped inner bark of the paper mulberry tree (*Broussonetia papyrifera*). The resulting paper is known as *gradaat saa*. To make a manuscript, sheets of this handmade paper are glued together to form a continuous rectangular sheet, folded into folios (pages) that open and shut like a concertina, described as *leporello*. The Horniman manuscript has a stiff protective cover made from sheets of mulberry paper glued together, lacquered, and stitched to the last folio. This is a relatively plain cover in comparison with many manuscripts that are lacquered and gilded. As I concluded later when the content was known, its subject matter did not warrant a decorative cover. When the manuscript was opened flat on the museum table, I counted eighty-seven folios on one side and the same number on the reverse side, making a total of one hundred and seventy-four folios. The manuscript is complete and in excellent condition. To find a Shan manuscript of this age in pristine condition was exciting, as until recently Shan manuscripts in Shan state were not well conserved. Most are kept in monasteries without any special storage facilities, subject to humidity and damage from insects such as white ants.

I put in a request for the manuscript to be photographed with a view to studying the content. Shan manuscripts are records of Buddhist doctrine and practice, but they also contain records of local history, creation myths, poetry, and folklore, treatises on law, herbalism, and supernatural remedies for illness. It would be a challenge to ascertain where the Horniman manuscript fitted among these categories, given that no scholars I consulted could read the script. There was one clue. The manuscript contained a set of geometric diagrams called *yantra* (mystical symbolic diagrams) generally associated with magico-religious ritual.

The Horniman manuscript is written in a script that evolved from earlier Shan scripts, dated to the thirteenth century.[5] Professor Sai Kam Mong has analysed the historical progression of Shan scripts from the sixteenth century to the present day. His book, *The History and Development of the Shan Scripts* (2004), contains illustrations of Shan scripts and demonstrates how the writing of consonants and vowels has evolved over time.

He claims that by the fourteenth century a form of Shan script was used in official government documents and diplomatic letters sent between Tai regional courts.[6] Shan was an irregular form of writing and was not systematised until 1949, long after the Horniman manuscript entered the collections. A degree of standardisation was introduced, and a modern script established. Extra vowels, tone marks, and consonants were added. The new script was formally adopted in 1955 and modified in 1975. The Horniman manuscript predates modern script by at least one hundred years.[7]

When I compared the scripts illustrated in Professor Sai's book with the Horniman manuscript, there are two types that appear similar. The shape of the letters and consonants and their arrangement suggests a derivation from Tai Yuan, a northern Tai script from Lan Na, and Tou Moan, a form of old Shan. According to Professor Sai, there are two versions of Yuan script, one for writing religious texts, the other for secular texts. Shan script and Tai Yuan script often appear in the same manuscript, particularly in treatises on

5. Report of the Secretary, Shan Phonology Commission, Hsipaw, 1974.

6. Sai Kam Mong, *The History and Development of the Shan Scripts*, Chiang Mai: Silkworm Books, 2004.

7. The Shan term for script is *lik*.

medicine and astrology. Other Shan experts who examined the manuscript identified some Burmese and Tai Khun letters.[8]

The task of finding a person who could read the script and translate it into modern Shan was a challenge. In 2010 I began a research project in northern Thailand and eastern Shan State focusing on healing rituals and ritual materials. I took a copy of the Horniman manuscript with me on field trips to eastern Shan State and to Chiang Rai and Tak in Thailand where many Shan people and Shan monks now live. I sought advice from local people about content and recognition of the script. Shan villagers said they were proud that the manuscript was considered important enough to be looked after in a prestigious museum in the UK. They described the script as 'magic language' and 'magic marks' and implied that only the *saya*, an expert in the arts of the supernatural, who originally owned the manuscript could read. I was not sure if they told me this because they were unable to read the script and therefore assumed it was magic language, or they were withholding information about the content because herbalism and supernatural remedies are secretive and not shared with outsiders. They were happy to provide information about the small number of mystical symbolic diagrams (*yantra*) included in the text. They told me they were talismans to protect against evil spirits, sets of letters and numbers placed in grids and formulated specifically to create good luck and to treat those possessed by evil spirits, manifested in physical and mental ill health.

In 2014 I published a book on Tai supernaturalism and included a few images from the Horniman manuscript to accompany the text.[9] I was determined to return to Shan State to solve the mystery of the 'magic language' and 'magic marks' spoken of by Shan villagers. Then, quite unexpectedly, I received an e-mail from Khun Tun Yee, an informant interviewed during my previous field trip. He had located two elderly

8. Tai inhabiting the central and eastern Shan State and part of Lan Na (north Thailand).

9. Susan Conway, *Tai Magic: Arts of the Supernatural*, Bangkok: River Books, 2014.

Shan experts, Long Te Za and Long Noi Na, who agreed to examine the manuscript and comment on the content. I e-mailed a photocopy. Several months later, Tun Yee responded. He began by telling me that Long Te Za and Long Noi Na said the folios were incorrectly numbered. Those labelled by the Horniman museum as eighty-eight to one hundred and seventy-four were, in fact, folios one to eighty-seven. In other words, the folios on the reverse side of the manuscript had been counted first by the curator who entered it in the records of the Horniman collection over a century and a half ago.

Long Te Za and Long Noi Na identified physical and mental ailments recorded in the text. They listed body paralysis, fever, blood disorders, lung and stomach complaints, skin wounds and skin infections, infertility, headaches, eye infections, and blindness. Mental illness was described as a condition caused by malignant ghosts and evil spirits. Each ailment they described was prefixed by either a healing Pali incantation or a magic spell (*katha*). to be chanted at the time a prescription was prepared and then repeated by the patient at the time it was taken. Long Te Za and Long Noi Na gave Tun Yee a verbal translation of *katha* spells which he wrote down and sent to me. They did not provide information on how ailments were treated. I was not sure if this was because such information was not in the text, or because they were unable to translate from a redundant script. Another possibility was they were observing the code of secrecy common among *saya*.

By the time I received the communication from Tun Yee, ten years had passed since the Horniman manuscript first came to light. Another four years would pass before further progress was made. It came in 2018 when I was approached in Oxford by Phra Dhammasami, Rector of the newly established Shan State Buddhist University. He asked if I was interested in teaching an MA course on anthropology and Shan material culture at the new university, which was situated in the Shan hills above the state capital Taunggyi. This was to be like the course I taught at the School of Oriental and African Studies in London. The offer presented an exciting challenge.

The start date was summer 2018. While packing academic material for the course, I included a copy of the Horniman manuscript, not because I expected any further translation would be possible but because it was a perfect example of how objects were conserved, catalogued, and stored in good museums, and how they were made available through accurate records for study by students today and in the future. I stress in my lectures the importance of conserving minority languages and scripts. Students need to understand how supressing and neglecting language and writing is a tool used to undermine the identity of minority peoples.

Teaching at Shan State Buddhist University presented an opportunity to support the study and conservation of Shan scripts through the creation of a digital library and conservation programme.[10] The library at Shan State Buddhist University has a new section set aside for the study of Shan manuscripts. Once the manuscripts donated by monasteries throughout Shan State have been cleaned, catalogued, and digitised they will be available for study worldwide. My programme of lectures at the university emphasised the link between manuscript texts and Shan culture, both religious and secular. I also underlined the importance of this new library as an example to other institutions in Shan State to accurately catalogue and conserve their collections.

At Shan State University, I met the abbot of the university, Phra Vicitta. During one of our meetings, I showed him a photocopy of the Horniman manuscript. He was interested in the content and contacted a distinguished *saya* who was a frequent visitor to the community. He agreed to help. My course ran for a full semester. As it came close to my departure, Phra Vicitta asked to see me. He was happy to present me with a translation of the Horniman text, typed into modern Shan. After years of speculating about the contents, this was a seminal moment. The mystery of the Shan manuscript stored for so long in a museum far away in London was a step

---

10. The Rockefeller Foundation provided a grant to support this project.

further to being solved. It would not be difficult to translate from modern Shan into English and easy to find a professional translator in Taunggyi.

The arrival of the Covid epidemic prevented this from happening. I left Taunggyi for Bangkok and on to London as an international shutdown was imposed. Communication became difficult. News was gleaned from Shan websites. Due to communication restrictions, it was not possible to have the manuscript translated in Taunggyi, but I was advised a Shan translator could be found in Chiang Mai, Thailand. I called a friend who contacted a professional Shan translator. She agreed to take on the work. The text was e-mailed to her and over a period of weeks she sent back the English translation. The contents of the manuscript she described as 'Medicines from Former Days'. Her translation, I realised, complemented the list of ailments and *katha* provided by Long Te Za and Long Noi Na. Ingredients included plant extracts, some cultivated, others gathered from the wild, animal extracts, and minerals. Some prescriptions contained polluted substances such as excrement and soil from cremation sites. It was clear that the Horniman manuscript provided remedies for healing and remedies for combating evil spirits using black magic.

The next questions to be solved were the date the manuscript was written and who authored it, bringing together herbal remedies and black magic, very different approaches to treatment. It is claimed that monks never practise black magic, they practise healing. A lay *saya* had to be involved. The answer was found in the text: 'This manuscript was written in the Tai Year Tao Yee in the fifth month on the eighth day by monk Mahathera Saokhimiya and saya Sao Silawan.'

Translating the date from Tao Yee years into the Buddhist Era and Christian Era presented two possibilities. The authors of the manuscript give the date according to the Chula Sakarat lunisolar calendar. It deciphers as either 2325 BE (1782 CE) or 2385 BE (1842 CE). In answer to the second question, a monk and *saya* collaborated in writing the text. That poses another question about collaboration and individual contributions. There are variations in handwriting on a few folios but not enough to provide a definitive answer.

Herbalism and magico-religious practices were passed orally from generation to generation long before they were written down. When they were written, it was by monks and laymen who had been monks because monasteries provided education for men. There was no formal education available to women.[11] However, herbalism and occult practices were not, and are not today, exclusively male. Women transferred knowledge orally, and there is a possibility that a few women learnt to read texts. Monasteries functioned like those in medieval England, male communities cultivating herbs and spices for ministering to the sick while offering prayers and rituals. Unlike Christian monks, it was relatively easy for Buddhist monks to leave the monastery and return to secular life. Most men entered the monastic life at some time in their lives, even if only as novices for three months, the period of Buddhist Lent. The movement between religious and secular life allowed knowledge about remedies and rituals for treating illness to pass from monastery to village and village to monastery. Although many probably forgot what they learnt in the monastery, short chants and healing remedies were easy to remember and useful at a practical level.

As the skills of black magic are highly secretive and rarely written down, it is interesting to note that the author, *saya* Sao Silawan, was prepared to list ingredients for black magic and his co-author, a monk, was prepared to accept the inclusion of such information. Does this indicate commonality in the way they were taught or similarity in the way they approached the act of healing? There are similarities in training. A lay *saya* serves an apprenticeship with an experienced *saya*. It can last up to ten years. In similar custom to Buddhist monks, he observes precepts. The five main precepts are no killing of a living object, no stealing, no falsehoods, no

11. Exceptions were those taught by missionaries and a few female members of the elite.

adultery, and no consumption of alcohol. Eight precepts add no food consumed after noon, no entertainment unless of a prescribed moral nature, and living without comfort by sitting on the floor during the day and sleeping on the floor at night. The more precepts the *saya* follows, the greater his power. This can increase through physical and mental endurance, for example, extensive painful tattooing on the face, arms, hands, torso, legs, and feet. Power also comes from ownership of ritual materials, including manuscripts. The following passage records an interview I conducted with a *saya* practising in Shan State:

> Maha Kaew is a charismatic man who became a saya without having family connections.... He studied with a master who taught him how to use ingredients to make magical prescriptions, as recorded in mulberry paper manuscripts passed down from generation to generation. Maha Kaew learnt incantations, magic spells, recipes for herbal medicines, and the power of yantra. To increase his power as a saya, he has been tattooed by thirty-two tattoo masters who worked layer upon layer until his skin became a blue-black colour except for areas around his eyes and nose, mouth, and soles of his feet.[12]

A well-established *saya* like Maha Kaew owns several manuscripts for reference and has learnt many *katha*. He spent time as a monk and learnt a few Pali healing incantations. Incantations and *katha* can both be chanted at the time prescriptions are prepared and when they are administered. *Saya* create altars (*khan kru*) and offer flowers, fruit, betel ingredients, and beeswax candles to the spirits. The altar may have statues of the Buddha and gods and goddesses like Nang Sulat Siwalee, protector of Buddhist scriptures; Nang Thorani, vanquisher of the demon god Mara; and Mae Phosop, patroness of rice culture.

12. Conway, *The Shan*, p. 174.

In the translation of *katha* provided by Long Te Za and Long Noi Na, each *katha* is matched to a disease. A *saya* chants *katha* to empower prescriptions. *Katha* are written and spoken in the local language, the equivalent of magic spells. When written down they appear as a mix of phrases, letters, symbols, and numbers in code. A *saya* gives directions to patients for healing rituals and a list of offerings to appease the spirits. In this manuscript, offerings are listed as red pennants, red flowers, red coloured biscuits, bananas, *paan* (a mixture of betel leaf, areca nut, and slaked lime), cutch, and tea. In contrast, a monk chants in Pali to call for protection and healing. The Pali in this manuscript is colloquial Pali, often described by monk scholars as 'incorrect'. It is used for incantations to the Triple Gem, the Buddha, the Dharma, and the Sangha and *sutta* (sacred texts), chanted to dispel evil spirits. In terms of offerings, monks prescribe ritual candles with *yantra* and containers of holy water.

Prescriptions make up most of the text in the Horniman manuscript. In 1910 the missionary Leslie Milne noted there was widespread knowledge of herbal remedies among men and women: 'There are several old men and women in each village, wise in spells and charms who have a considerable knowledge of the virtues of certain kinds of barks and herbs.'[13]

Ingredients were grown in home and monastery gardens or gathered in the forest and sold on stalls in local markets. The text stipulates ingredients be gathered and processed on auspicious days. Women who controlled market stalls in Shan State were purveyors of many ingredients listed in these prescriptions. Writing in 1837, over twenty years before the date the manuscript entered the collections of the Horniman Museum, the British explorer Captain McCleod wrote: 'In the bazar I saw many medicinal roots.'[14]

13. Leslie Milne and Wilbur Willis Cochrane, *Shans at Home*, reprint New York: Paragon, 1910, p. 178.

14. Volker Grabowsky and Andrew Turton, eds., *The Gold and Silver Road of Trade and Friendship: The McLeod and Richardson Diplomatic Missions to Tai States in 1837*, Chiang Mai: Silkworm Books, 2003, p. 383.

Animal extracts came mostly from wild animals hunted in local forests. They and their habitats were plentiful in nineteenth-century Shan State. McLeod noted deer horn and rhinoceros horn for sale in Shan markets. Deer horn was believed to keep the kidneys and spleen healthy, strengthen bones and muscles, and promote blood flow.[15] Rhino horn was mixed with herbal ingredients for treating fever or relieving the symptoms of arthritis and gout. It was also believed to cure headaches, hallucinations, high blood pressure, typhoid, snakebite, food poisoning, and possession by spirits. The claim that rhino horn was prescribed as an aphrodisiac is contested.[16] McLeod also lists bears, tigers, pangolins, porcupines, and pythons hunted for their skins and internal organs. Bear bile was used to reduce fever, to heal inflammation, and for pain reduction. It is recorded as a treatment for liver disease, haemorrhoids, heat convulsions, and epilepsy. Ground tiger bone was for healing ulcers and burns and to cure typhoid, malaria, dysentery, and rheumatism. Its whiskers and teeth were worn as talismans to protect against illness. Pangolins were hunted for their scales that were dried and roasted and used to treat malaria and deafness, certain nervous conditions, and women possessed by evil spirits. Porcupines were captured for bezoar, a stony secretion extracted from the stomach and a cure for digestive ailments and dengue fever. Python's bones, gall bladder and skin were treatment for rheumatism, headache, and diabetes, and ailments caused by evil spirits. Stick lac, a secretion of insects, treated liver damage.

Other ingredients listed in the manuscript include alum crystals, ground to a fine powder and used to treat open wounds and sores. Grass from local termite nests is also listed. Termites were widely used in traditional

15. Chen L., Wang X., and Huang B. J., 'The Genus Hippocampus: A Review on Traditional Medicinal Uses, Chemical Constituents, and Pharmacological Properties', *Journal of Ethnopharmacology*, 2015, 162: 104–11.

16. 16 Jeremy Hsu, 'The Hard Truth about the Rhino Horn', *Scientific American*, 5 April 2017.

medicine in Southeast Asia for treating fungal and bacterial infections.[17] A specific termite hill could acquire a reputation for good luck, so a piece of soil or grass from a termite hill was thought to aid the healing process. One of the prescriptions involves burning an ant's nest and gathering the ash as a treatment for lesions. In terms of imported ingredients, long-distance traders from Burma brought kerosene (in translation 'crude oil'), used to treat sores and wounds.[18] Shan trade with China included honey, a remedy for healing wounds.

Although the Horniman manuscript contains a comprehensive list of illnesses and prescriptions they are not arranged in any order, in this publication, for the sake of clarity, the text has been organised into chapters. The first chapter gives prescriptions with ingredients for making pills that are given orally or ground up with other ingredients. It also includes prescriptions where fresh ingredients are used without the addition of ready-made pills. The second chapter contains mystical symbolic diagrams (*yantra*) and explains how they are used in healing and as mechanisms for protection. The third chapter contains magic spells (*katha*, translated with the help of *saya* Long Te Za and *saya* Long Noi Na and Khun Tun Yee.

It has not been possible to translate into English all the ingredients given in these prescriptions because some names are in local dialect not understood today. Sometimes the translation of a plant name into English does not match a species likely to have been available in Asia in the nineteenth century. For example, a plant translated from Shan as 'pink wonder' means in English a type of daffodil that grows in the cool climate of northern Europe. 'Pink wonder' must be a vernacular term for another plant that grows in Shan State.

17. Rob Verpoorte, 'Food and Medicine: Old Traditions, Novel Opportunities', *Journal of Ethnobiology and Ethnomedicine*, 2015, 11: 29.

18. Leslie Milne and Wilbur Willis Cochrane, *Shans at Home*, reprint New York: Paragon, 1970.

Collecting herbs is linked to phases of the moon and power attributed to each phase. Simple diagrams available in a Shan market chart four main phases and illustrate with a scale of marks the power held in each phase. Herbs harvested at full moon when power is strong have the greatest healing power. The full moon of November is the most powerful. Some herbalists restrict the collection of herbs only to the night of a full moon. Power is particularly strong at times of solar and lunar eclipses, when the plant world is believed to be particularly charged.[19] The female herbalist Nang Lord, who is practising today, confirmed the importance of collecting on auspicious days, as recorded in an interview with her:

> Nang Lord runs a successful herbal medicine practice. One basic ingredient is wild honey that she collects on auspicious days, calculated according to a lunar calendar.... Before beginning to make potions and ointments, she offers the honey to the spirits for a blessing. It is blended with dried and ground herbs, up to ten different types for each batch. She also distils herbs into soap-like cakes that are used in cleansing rituals and as a soothing wash for babies and small children that cry a lot. Nang Lord does not divulge the secrets of her recipes although she admits to using plants with auspicious names and choosing others for their physical characteristics.[20]

As Nang Lord admits, the main purpose of collecting herbs is medicinal, but some are gathered for other reasons. She gathers plants with specific physical characteristics. A 'strong' plant that grows upright with robust stems is an ingredient because the attribute of strength can pass to a patient to help recovery from illness. She includes other plants considered to be auspicious. For example, the sacred water lily (*Nelumbo nucifera*) a symbol

---

19. B. J. Terwiel, *Monks and Magic*, Bangkok: White Lotus, 1994, p. 225.
20. Conway, *Tai Magic*, pp. 180–3.

of purity, enlightenment, and rebirth aids recovery. Nang Lord does not use plants with names associated with pollution, for example, asafoetida (*Ferula apiaceae*), known as 'devil's dung'. It is included among ingredients listed in the Horniman manuscript.

Prescriptions in this manuscript indicate a different approach to treating illness than in Western medical practice. Less emphasis is placed on homogenous forms of diagnosis, the name of a disease, its origin, and pre-set forms of treatment. The Shan practitioner relies on practical knowledge of plants and personal experience of what works best for individual patients. It is a form of treatment not standardised and is difficult for Western doctors to monitor. As one herbalist explains: 'The important thing is not what you call a disease or from where it comes but rather to know which preparation must be used to get rid of it.'[21]

---

21. Viggo Brun and Trond Schumacher, *Traditional Herbal Medicine in Northern Thailand*, Bangkok: White Lotus, 1994, pp. 209–10.

Folios 1–4

Chapter 1

PRESCRIPTIONS FOR MAKING PILLS

1. Prescriptions with Ingredients for Making Pills

Pills are prepared in batches. Barend Terwiel, who in 1965 served time as an ordained monk at Wat Sanchao, a monastery near the town of Ratchaburi, saw their production in a monastic community: 'There are some older monks who are famous for the healing power of their pills, manufactured from ground up sacred objects. Others have a regular clientele for their bundles of herbs from which the patient may brew a medicinal tea.'[1] Terwiel revised the text in 1991 and 1992 while teaching in Southeast Asia. Much of it remains relevant today.

The reference to 'ground up sacred objects' points to section four of this chapter, controlling evil spirits, ghosts, and witches with treatments that use black magic. Sacred objects for grinding are identified as in proximity to a Buddhist source. They include wood shavings from a monastery door, chips from floor tiles laid near a Buddha image, and ground fragments of a monk's alms bowl.

---

1. B. J. Terwiel, *Monks and Magic: An Analysis of Religious Ceremonies in Central Thailand*, Bangkok: White Lotus, 1994.

Recipe One

The first recipe has over fifty plant ingredients plus rhino blood, pangolin liver, bear bile, and porcupine bezoar, and the chemicals alum and green vitriol crystal. The standard weight for ingredients is given as 4.08233 grams (63 grains).

Method

Grind a small rhizome of ginger, galangal, stone ginger, rosy leadwort, black cumin, wild ginger, false daisy, red entada bean (snuffbox sea bean), devil's tree bark, rhino blood, liver from a pangolin, leaves from a dog bush, mustard seeds, asafoetida (devil's dung), nutgall black seed, roots from a drumstick tree, black turmeric, sweet flag, black entatda bean (snuffbox sea bean black), elephant ear plant (also called night-scented lily), willow-leaved shrimp plant, Malabar nut, white turmeric root, milk hedge leaves, Chinese ginger, white seed of Indian or Jamaican wild liquorice, porcupine bezoar (a stony secretion which forms in a porcupine's stomach), a shallot, chamber bitter, nutmeg, mace, cloves, green milkweed climber, heart-leaved moonseed, also called guduchi, papaya tree root, Indian ginseng root, winter cherry, bowing lady tuber root, mango seed, pinewood, long pepper root, fennel, anise, cumin, dill, golden shower tree bark, fever nut, alum, green vitriol crystal, white dammar tree sap, tamarind seed, and bear bile. Grind ingredients into a paste and cut into circular shaped pills.

Recipe Two

The second recipe contains over forty plant ingredients plus porcupine quill, cowrie shell, and black salt. The recipe stipulates that one ingredient, alfalfa grass, must be taken from a termite hill. Each ingredient weighs 08233 grams (63 grains).

Method

Grind curry leaves, croton root, yellow cinnabar, black salt, wireweed, Indian ipecac, cotton seed, fruit of sugar palm, Java bean, dog bush, tagara, lemon basil, stink vine root, root of alfalfa grass growing on a termite hill, root and bark of Indian ivy rue, grey leaf heliotrope, aromatic ginger, golden thread vine, porcupine quills, tea leaves, bitter snake gourd, black bean root, candy lily, bitter oleander, Japanese yam, pomegranate bush root, croton, cowrie shell, peel from a chestnut, shoot from a giant reed, fiddlehead fern root, young white willow, wild asparagus, rough chaff tree bark, root of the common bush weed, honeysuckle, seed from a jackfruit fallen from a tree, lemon vine, root cinnamon, and shikakai bark. Add water to make a paste and cut into circular pills.

Recipe Three

The third recipe contains over twenty plant ingredients plus a wasp's nest, the gall bladder of a python, sal ammoniac, and sugar. Each ingredient weighs 4.08233 grams (63 grains).

Method

Grind together fragrant bay leaves, Indian bay seed, blue fountain bush, mistletoe growing on a jackfruit tree, sweet flag, pipe vine, Indian birthwort, coriander seed, neem, extract from a wasp's nest, black sesame root, black chili root, quince seed, lime tree root, giant fern tree, gall bladder from a python, fragrant anneslea, brown love grass, rain tree leaves, Indian bay leaves, Chinese laurel leaves, red sandalwood, bitter cucumber, chaulmoongra, sal ammoniac and sugar. Add water to make a paste and cut into circular pills.

Recipe Four

The fourth recipe contains five plant ingredients plus deer horn and honey. In this recipe the tical is used as a measure (one tical equals 16.3293 grams).

Method

Prepare 7.5 ticals of asafoetida, 2 ticals of Indian snake root, 4 ticals of mat daisy, 20 ticals of deer horn, 5 ticals of black cardamom, and 30 ticals of honey. Grind ingredients together with a little water to make a paste and cut into circular pills.

Recipe Five

In recipe five, pills are concocted for the specific purpose of protection against evil spirits and demons. There are fifteen plant ingredients plus a mix of tiger, python, and vulture gall bladders.

Method

Grind zebrawood, oak apple or oak gall, asafoetida, nutmeg, cloves, black bean root, Himalayan gentian, rosy leadwort, five kinds of *umbelliferae* (fennel, anise or sweet fennel, cumin, black cumin, dill), and pepper. Mix with the gall bladder of a tiger, a vulture, and a python. Form the paste into round pills. Take the prescribed number of pills with water that is purposefully thrown up onto the roof of a house and collected as it runs down from the roof.

Recipe Six

Recipe six creates pills that protect against witchcraft and demons. There are fifteen plant ingredients.

Method

Grind together lemongrass, giant elephant ear plant (night-scented lily), blackberry lily or candy lily, small rhizome ginger, 7 chilies, 7 purging croton, sweet flag, entada bean (snuffbox sea bean), five kinds of *umbelliferae* (fennel, anise or sweet fennel, cumin, black cumin, dill), dog bush, and dodder or golden thread vine. Form the mixture into rounded pills. Swallow one pill. Use a second pill to rub around the inside of the mouth and over the lips and eyelids.

2. Prescriptions that Include Pills Ground up with Other Ingredients

In this section illnesses are treated with a mix of ground pills, herbs, and oils. Three pills are the most common number although one prescription requires seven pills. They are crushed with other ingredients and dissolved in water for taking orally or mixed in oil to make lotions and compresses and for massage oil. Where pills are crushed as part of these prescriptions, it is not clear from the text which of the six types (see above) is being used in each recipe. This may be intentional as *saya* were often secretive about recipe details.

Digestive Disorders

For indigestion, gas pains, a knotted feeling in the abdomen, bloating, and cramps, grind 3 pills into powder and dissolve in an infusion made from boiled roots of the blue fountain bush and the silk tree.

For burping and passing gas, take 3 pills ground together with pepper, sesame oil, and mustard oil.

For food poisoning, take 3 pills dissolved in the foam formed as water spills over the top of a terrace in a rice field.

For stomach pains, grind 7 ticals (114.3051 grams) of ginger, 7 ticals of turmeric, and 7 pills into a fine powder. Dissolve in warm water and drink.

Heart, Lung, and Circulatory Disorders

For an abnormally fast heartbeat accompanied by a fever, dissolve 3 pills in an infusion made from boiled golden shower seeds.

For the symptoms of asthma, chew 3 pills together with 3 young shoots of the Malabar nut tree. Wash down with warm water.

For poor circulation resulting in cold hands and feet, mix 4.08233 grams (63 grains) of lime with 3 pills ground into a fine powder. Sprinkle the powder on crushed garlic and spread on pear leaves and red castor bean leaves. Heat the leaves over a live charcoal fire. Apply the baked leaves to the palms of the hands and soles of the feet.

Abnormal Bleeding

For bleeding in the mouth and throat, dissolve 3 pills in an ointment made from pepper, small rhizome ginger, and roots of the drumstick tree.

For rectal bleeding or bleeding from the sex organs, grind 3 pills with salt and pepper and dissolve in warm water. Apply to the affected area.

Fevers

For a sensation of heat followed by chills and a feeling of being generally unwell, take 3 pills with lime water.

For a fever, dissolve 3 pills in a liquid made from boiled Java beans and false daisy.

For a fever with a headache and symptoms of fatigue and insomnia, grind 3 pills into powder and dissolve in an infusion made from boiled roots of the blue fountain bush and the silk tree.

Body Aches and Rheumatism

For aching hands and feet, grind 3 pills with oil from ambergris and rub on the joints at the wrist and ankles.

For pain in the feet, make a lotion from 3 pills ground with earth from a termite mound and water in which rice has been soaked. Use as a massage lotion.

For aching thighs, grind 3 pills with alcohol and use as a massage lotion.

For back pain and aches extending along the spine, take 3 pills dissolved in a liquid made from boiled down small ginger rhizomes. Apply and massage gently on the back.

For swollen, bruised, and cold feet, make a lotion from 3 ground pills and lemon juice. Massage gently into the joints.

Urinary Tract Disorders

For urinary retention, grind together on a wetted flat, stone mango seeds, pinewood seeds, and seeds taken from a plant 'growing on an outdoor veranda'. Grind until a pulpy consistency is reached. Take with 3 pills washed down with water collected from runoff from the roof of a house. The runoff must be intentionally created by throwing water up on the roof three times.

Wound Infections

For infected wounds, grind 3 pills with the sap of a freshly harvested banana tree trunk and crude oil (kerosene) to create a pulp. Apply the pulp around the wound, avoiding the actual lesion.

Headaches and Dizziness

For headaches and dizziness, take 3 pills mixed with small rhizome ginger, false daisy, and a little sesame oil.

Numbness and Loss of Taste

For numbness in the mouth and throat and a loss of taste, grind 3 pills and mix with crude oil (kerosene). Use as drops in the mouth and on the tongue. Leave 'for a while' and then scrape off.

Mental Instability

For a fever accompanied by symptoms of hysteria caused by spells attributed to negative supernatural power, grind to a pulpy consistency 3 pills and the roots of wireweed. Add water and take as a drink. This pulp can also be used as a calming body massage lotion.

3. Prescriptions with Ingredients Excluding Pills

The prescriptions in this section are a mix of herbs, animal and human extracts, and minerals. They treat a similar range of diseases as listed in sections one and two with the addition of those caused specifically by the action of evil spirits. Evil spirits can magically introduce foreign substances into the body. One prescription treats earache caused by an insect magically inserted into the ear. Dog excrement is an ingredient to appease evil spirits that eat excrement. Ash from burnt human and animal bone treats swollen lymph glands caused by evil spirts who introduce foreign bodies into glands. Mental instability presents as hysteria and insanity caused by possession and is treated with a purgative to help the body expel evil spirits from the body and a body rub made from pork fat, a polluted ingredient that appeases evil spirits.

One remedy treats a disease described in the text as 'mad cow disease'. This definition challenges some concepts of a disease that in the West is seen as a twentieth-century discovery, first diagnosed in the United Kingdom. Mad cow disease referred to in this manuscript is a disease that can be traced back to the fifth century BC.[2] It is probably this form or a variant that infected Shan livestock. No symptoms are given in the text, but it is described as a fatal disease. The prescription for treatment includes condensed milk. Condensed milk, as understood in Western culinary circles, means a form

---

2. V. McAlister, 'Sacred Disease of Our Times: Failure of the Infectious Disease Model of Spongiform Encephalopathy', *Clinical and Investigative Medicine*, 2005, 28(3): 101–4.

of milk first produced in Europe in 1820. It is unlikely that it was available in early nineteenth-century Shan State. There is an alternative source. Writing in the thirteenth century, Marco Polo noted that the Tatars condensed milk into paste and reconstituted it with water. The Tatar method for condensing milk was known to societies in Southeast Asia and is the likely ingredient in this prescription.

Mineral components include arsenic trisulphide, used in the West to treat *herpes zosta*, usually known as shingles. Here arsenic trisulphide is part of the treatment for swollen lymph nodes, kidney stones, and paralysis. Green vitriol treats iron deficiency, and in these prescriptions is an ingredient for curing toothache, earache, paralysis, and insanity. Opium can cause constipation so is an effective treatment for cholera, dysentery, and diarrhoea. As a cough suppressant, opium treats bronchitis, tuberculosis, and other respiratory illnesses. In the nineteenth century, opium was used to treat nervous disorders due to its sedative and tranquilising properties. In these prescriptions, it is an ingredient for treating fever and heat prostration and pain caused by kidney stones and haemorrhoids. It is also prescribed for rheumatism and insomnia.

Digestive Disorders

For vomiting, grind together blackberry lily or candy lily roots, Indian ginseng roots, croton roots, and black roots of alfalfa grass. Dissolve in warm water and take as a drink.

For a bloated painful stomach, grind pepper with small ginger rhizome, 17 grains of rice, 7 Indian jujube leaves, 7 Indian wild pepper leaves, and 3 parts lime extract. Dissolve in warm water and drink. An alternative prescription for a bloated stomach involves grinding wild ginger, small ginger rhizome, and false daisy together. Dissolve in warm water and drink.

For sharp stabbing pains in the abdomen, grind Himalayan gentian, rosy leadwort, black cumin, and small rhizome ginger together. Dissolve in warm water and drink.

A second prescription for stabbing pains in the abdomen, grind black cumin, rosy leadwort, dog bush, pepper, wild ginger, turmeric, ginger rhizome, Indian wild pepper, and coriander seeds together and take orally.

A third prescription for stabbing pains in the abdomen, grind chamber bitter, yellow turmeric, wild ginger, asafoetida (devil's dung), nutmeg, cloves, pepper, black cumin, and arsenic trisulphide and take orally.

For flatulence, boil small ginger rhizomes with devil's tree bark. Take the infusion as a drink.

For burping and passing gas and discomfort in the abdomen, squeeze juice from green milkweed climber and heart-leaved moonseed and mix with pepper and small ginger rhizome. Take orally.

A second prescription for gas, grind together black cumin, pepper, sap from the white dammar tree, and catechu from an acacia tree. Add rhino blood. Take orally.

A third prescription for gas pains, grind together asafoetida, Indian wild pepper, coriander seeds, pepper, nutgall black seed, purging croton, sweet flag, black ginger, red entada bean, black entada bean, night-scented lily, and false daisy. Take orally.

For stomach pain caused by gas experienced in the daytime and at night, grind together papaya tree bark, pepper, small ginger rhizome, and Indian gooseberry. Dissolve in warm water. Take as a drink.

A second prescription for gas pains in the stomach, roots of bayan fig, roots of Indian wild pepper, roots of white willow tree, roots of vine-like fern or Japanese climbing fern, black nightshade, roots of bitter gourd, and pepper. Boil all the ingredients together, strain and drink the liquid.

For stomach cramps and a knotted feeling in the abdomen, mix rhino blood with pangolin liver and pepper and take orally.

A second prescription for stomach cramps, grind together galangal, small ginger rhizome, leaves of milk hedge, nutgall black seed, Chinese ginger, pepper, white seed of Indian or Jamaican wild liquorice, asafoetida, porcupine bezoars, and shallots. Dissolve in warm water and drink.

A third prescription for stomach cramps, grind together sweet flag, asafoetida, rosy leadwort, pepper, shallot, and galangal with tiger meat. Dissolve in warm water and drink.

A fourth prescription for stomach cramps, grind together 25 ticals (408.233 grams) of tamarind, Indian gooseberry, and small rhizome ginger, 5 ticals (81.6465 grams) of false daisy and kassod, 1 tical (16.3293 grams) of ash from the middle of a fire, pepper, and 'odoriferous medicinal salt' (black salt). Dissolve in warm water and take orally.

For general gas pains, grind to a powder fennel, anise or sweet fennel, cumin, black cumin, dill, nutmeg, cloves, dog bush, long pepper, pepper, Himalayan gentian, white sandalwood, asafoetida, onion, fragrant bay, galangal, small rhizome ginger, wild ginger, elephant ear plants (night-scented lily), ginger, and aromatic ginger. Add rhino blood and swallow with water.

For general stomach pain, mix wild ginger, pepper, and small rhizome ginger together and dissolve in water. Take as a drink.

For hiccups, grind rosy leadwort with roots of the moringa tree. Dissolve in the liquid drained from boiled rice. Warm the mixture and drink.

For stomach spasms, grind together white turmeric root, roots of bowing lady flower, seeds of wild ginger, and rosy leadwort. Mix with sugar and honey and dissolve in water. Take as a drink.

For inflammation of the stomach and small intestine, grind together 8.16466 grams of black cumin, 8.16466 grams of tamarind, 8.16466 grams of Indian gooseberry tree bark with 7 peppercorns, 7 long peppers, 8.16466 grams of dry roasted salt, and 3 pods of cardamom. Dissolve in warm water and drink.

For a laxative, grind together the root of Indian ginseng, roots and fruit of purging croton, rosy leadwort, pepper, long pepper, arsenic trisulphide, green vitriol, alum, and opium. Dilute in warm water and drink.

For blood in the stool, grind together Indian ginseng, flaming lily, pepper, long pepper, and cardamom. Dissolve in water and take as a drink.

For pain around the belly button, grind sweet flag, Chinese ginger root, black cumin, and mustard seeds. Apply to the skin in the belly button area.

For a purgative, grind to a powder 5 ticals of nutgall seed, 5 ticals of red roots of the red rex begonia vine, 5 ticals of bark from the golden shower tree, 5 ticals of seed pod of shikakai, and 5 ticals purging croton fruits. Take orally.

For appendicitis and pain around the belly button, grind devil's horsewhip, 7 tobacco plant leaves, and 7 shoots of elephant grass. Boil together in water, strain, and take as a drink.

Heart Conditions and Blood Pressure

For a feeling of pressure and pain in the chest, grind baked red entada beans together with pepper and small ginger rhizome. Dissolve in water and take as a drink.

A second prescription for chest pain, grind white sandalwood, red sandalwood, silver ore, and galena (lead ore) on a grinding stone with water in which rice has been soaked to create a pulpy mixture. Strain the liquid and take orally.

A third prescription for chest pain, grind red entada bean, pepper, and small rhizome ginger together to a powder. Dilute in water and take as a drink.

A fourth prescription for chest pain, grind willow-leaved shrimp plant, Malabar nut, wild ginger, small ginger rhizome, black cumin, and pepper. Mix with rhino blood. Dissolve in warm water and drink.

For blood pressure and chest pain, grind black cumin, pepper, small ginger rhizome, and shallot together into a powder. Dissolve in water and drink.

Eye Conditions

For inflammation of the eyelids, boil down in a copper pot of water, nutmeg, cloves, green vitriol, black myrobalan, tea fruit [sic], tamarind, and 7 grains of dry roasted sticky rice. Apply on the eyelids.

For blurred vision, take 7 pomegranate leaves, 7 young shoots of soap pods, and 7 young shoots of Indian gooseberry. Put in a copper pot of water and boil down. To create a pulpy paste, add green vitriol, red sandalwood, and nutmeg. Use as an eye ointment.

For inflammation of the eye, mix extract of goat gall bladder with goat milk and human milk. Use as eye drops.

Earache

For pain relief when an insect is trapped in the ear, grind dog excrement with mugwort. Wrap and tie the mixture inside a black cloth. Immerse in a pot of boiling water. Remove the cloth and drink the liquid with pepper water.

Flu Symptoms

For laryngitis, flu with a sore throat, and loss of voice, mix Himalayan gentian, pepper, black cumin, long pepper, nutmeg, cloves, Chinese ginger, wild ginger, 2.04117 grams of burnt earth turned over by a plough, 2.04117 grams of earth from a fish trap basket, and 2.04117 grams of cow dung as applied on the walls of a rice granary. Add 2.04117 grams of pepper, bitter bottle gourd, and holy basil. Grind to a powder and mix with a clear solution of lime dissolved in water. Swallow in one go.

Headaches

For a dull and heavy head, mix wild ginger, Indian wild pepper, and pepper together. Drink with water. If the ingredients are mixed and left dry, the powder can be used as snuff.

For headache and drowsiness, grind together salt, Indian wild pepper, pepper, a section taken from a wasp's nest, ash from a fireplace, and 7 grains of rice taken from among grains trapped in the cracks of a wooden pestle and mortar. Dissolve in water and drink.

For female headaches, mix black cumin, roots of alfalfa grass, and ash from a fireplace. Use as an inhalant.

For headaches, make an ointment to rub on the forehead using ground white turmeric, elephant ear leaves from the night-scented lily, aromatic ginger, dog bush, wild ginger, sweet flag, fragrant bay, cinnamon, and sacred garlic pear.

Skin Disorders

For pimples, grind the roots of Indian ginseng or winter cherry, roots of bowing lady flower, or the stems and roots of giant bamboo. Grind on a grinding stone. Add water in which rice has been soaked and mix with the other ingredients to a pulpy consistency. Apply on the surface of the pimples.

For a skin eruption, grind white seed of Indian wild liquorice and sugarcane on a grinding stone to create a pulpy mix. Apply to the skin in the affected area.

For a large pimple (a boil), grind white seeds of Indian wild liquorice, wild asparagus, sparrow's droppings, walnuts, wild bean, and yellow pumpkin on a grinding stone with water in which rice has been soaked to create a pulpy mix. Apply to the affected area.

Serious Skin Lesions (possibly made by a tiger)

Take an ant's nest from a tree and burn it. Gather the ash and apply to the scratches.

Toothache

For toothache, grind together pepper, Indian wild pepper, nutmeg, cloves, green vitriol, alum, peel of bael fruit or stone apple, and strychnine. Apply to the affected tooth.

Swollen Lymph Nodes

For swollen painful lymph nodes in the groin, collect the ash from the tripod that supports a cooking pot over the fire and grind together with 7 mistletoe plants, ash from the burnt wood of a bed support, and ash from an old burnt chair. Apply to the groin area. If this remedy does not cure the condition, try the next remedy.

A second prescription for swollen painful lymph nodes in the groin, burn a human bone, a black chicken's bone, a sparrow bone, and a buffalo bone. Grind the ashes to a powder and apply to the groin area.

A third prescription for swollen painful lymph nodes in the groin area, grind cloves, nutmeg, and arsenic trisulphide together to a powder and drink with water cooled from a steaming pot.

Poor Circulation

For trembling, cold hands, squeeze juice from *paan* (a mix of betel leaf, areca nut and slaked lime), add pepper and a pinch of salt. Take orally or use to rub on the hands and feet.

For numbness in the hands and feet caused by cold weather, grind purging croton, chili, leaves of Indian ginseng or winter cherry, Indian wild pepper, and rosy leadwort. Take orally in water or use as a lotion rubbed on the hands and feet.

For muscle strain, grind seeds of Indian ginseng or winter cherry, tamarind seeds, Indian jujube fruit, sugar palm fruit, and fruit of Ceylon oak to a powder. Take orally.

A second prescription for muscle strain, grind Indian sarsaparilla, small ginger rhizome, cardamom, seven grains of rice, seven peppercorns, and one purging croton fruit together. Dissolve in water and drink.

For painful sprains, boil together in a pot 7 dog bush leaves, Siam weed or Christmas bush leaves, croton, needle wood tree, cinnamon, wild asparagus, and pepper. Strain the liquid and drink.

For stiffness in the muscles, muscle cramp, a knot-like feeling in the muscles, and 'muscle displacement' [*sic*], mix white lime quarried from limestone, wild ginger, ash from the middle of a fireplace, Indian wild pepper, small rhizome ginger, Chinese ginger roots, long pepper, and black cumin. Add warm water and apply as a massage or body rub.

For arthritis, grind croton, dog bush, tobacco, yellow turmeric, wild ginger, and black cumin. Add warm water and use as a massage or body rub.

For stiffness in the body, grind to a powder 10 ticals (163.293 grams) of bael fruit or stone apple, 10 ticals of crooked rough bush (aspen) or 10 ticals of toothbrush tree, 10 ticals of wild asparagus, 10 ticals of croton, 10 ticals of grey nicker, 10 ticals of roots of freshwater mangrove, 10 ticals of golden shower tree, 10 ticals of pepper, 10 ticals of long pepper, 5 ticals of sweet flag, 1 tical of nutmeg, 1 tical of cloves, 5 ticals of *umbelliferae* (fennel, anise or sweet fennel, cumin, black cumin or dill), 1 tical blackberry lily or 5 ticals candy lily, and 5 ticals wild ginger. Dissolve in water and take as a drink every evening.

For rheumatic pains, grind together beehive ginger, Chinese ginger, sweet flag, wild ginger, orchid root, rosy leadwort, Himalayan gentian, Siamese cassia buds, roots of a candy lily, roots of red castor bean plants, and roots from a drumstick tree. Dissolve the powder in water and take orally.

A second prescription for rheumatism (also treats haemorrhoids and inflammation of the stomach and small intestine), grind together 8.16466 grams black cumin, 8.16466 grams tamarind, 8.16466 grams of bark from an Indian gooseberry tree, 7 peppercorns, 7 long pepper, 8.16466 grams dry roasted salt, and 3 pods of cardamom. Dissolve in warm water and take as a drink.

To relieve stiffness in the neck and back, and back pain, grind together white turmeric root, red turmeric, yellow turmeric, woolly dyeing rosebay, and sweet indrajao. Take orally.

A second prescription for stiffness, grind together 1 tical of mat daisy, ¼ tical of asafoetida, 1 tical of long pepper, 1 tical of nutmeg, 1 tical of monkey fruit or monkey jack, and 8 ticals of honey. Take the medicine orally every morning and evening.

Fevers, Dehydration, and Heat Prostration

For a fever, grind to a powder nutmeg, cloves, fennel, anise, sweet fennel, cumin, black cumin, dill, pepper, asafoetida, opium, white seeds of Indian or Jamaican wild liquorice, grey nicker seed, Indian bay, climbing wattle, curry leaves, cardamom, and Indian wild pepper. Add the bear bile with warm water. Take as a drink. This potion can also be used as a body rub.

A second prescription for a fever, mix dog bush, sweet basil, pepper, and asafoetida together and dissolve in warm water as a drink.

A third prescription for a fever, grind fresh Indian gooseberry, nutmeg, cloves, black cumin, aromatic ginger, sweet flag, and pepper. Dissolve in warm water and drink.

A fourth prescription for a fever, grind bitter bottle gourd seeds, lemon basil, and bark of the Indian trumpet tree together. Mix the powder with sesame oil and take orally.

For a high fever, grind leaves of a drooping fig plant, dissolve in rice water and take as a drink.

For lowering body temperature, mix black cumin, white seed of Indian or Jamaican wild liquorice, porcupine bezoars, and shallots. Dissolve in warm water and drink.

To cure a high fever caused by cholera, mix asafoetida, opium, small ginger rhizome, wild ginger, ground porcupine quill, and golden thread vine. Grind together and dissolve in warm water. Take as a drink. This concoction can also be used as a body rub.

A second prescription to reduce a fever caused by cholera, grind turmeric root, 7 roots of alfalfa grass growing on a termite hill, and roots of paper mulberry. Dissolve in water and drink.

For heat prostration, grind sweet flag, devil's horsewhip, dodder or gold thread vine, turmeric, wild pepper, and asafoetida together. Dissolve in warm water and drink.

Another prescription for heat prostration with symptoms of loss of taste and a numb feeling in the mouth and throat (described as 'symptoms that can be fatal'), grind together 272.155 grams of opium, 272.155 grams of salt, and 544.31grams of gold thread vine together. Take orally. This can also be used as a body rub.

For heat stress (defined as 'inside the body'), mix long pepper, nutgall black seed, and black cumin together. Dissolve in warm water and drink.

For sores and swelling of the tongue and mouth caused by heat stress, leading to difficulties in speaking, grind nutmeg, cloves, black cumin, grey nicker, bitter bottle gourd seeds, and lemon basil together with oil. The mixture is applied directly to the sores in the mouth and on the tongue.

Delirium

Grind together pepper, black cumin, long pepper, blackberry lily or candy lily, black turmeric, beehive ginger, Chinese ginger root, root for wild ginger, and soot from the fire. Add warm water and take as a drink.

Urinary Problems, Kidney Stones, and Sex Problems

For urinary retention, grind pomegranate roots that are growing towards the east with 7 peppercorns. Add a little sesame oil and boil in water in which rice has been soaked. Take as a drink.

A second prescription for urinary retention, grind the bark of the golden shower tree, orchid tree, and dried ginger together with 1 tical (16.3293 grams) of croton and 3 purging croton seeds. Dissolve in water and take as a drink.

For kidney stones and stones lodged in the urinary tract, grind together nutmeg, cloves, black cumin, arsenic trisulphide, tortoiseshell, cowrie shell, opium, mustard seeds, Indian wild pepper leaves, and young leaves of purging croton. Dissolve in warm water and take as a drink.

A second prescription for kidney stones, grind together cowrie shell, white seeds of Indian wild liquorice, wild asparagus, and peel from a ridge gourd. Dilute in water in which rice has been soaked. Take as a drink.

For haematuria (blood in the urine) suffered by men and women, collect yellow damson roots that grow towards the west and mix with devil's horsewhip. Boil down from three parts water until one part water. Take as a drink.

For frequency, boil a section taken from a mango tree trunk in water. Strain and drink the liquid.

A second prescription for frequency, boil common bush weed in water. Strain and drink the liquid.

For a shrinking penis, take white wonder or white turmeric roots, and black chili root. Cover in water and boil. Take the liquid as a drink and rub the liquid onto the affected area.

Syphilis

Grind Indian ipecac, Himalayan gentian, and black cumin together and add warm water. Take as a drink and rub on the affected areas.

Diabetes

Grind rosy leadwort, cinnamon seeds, fragrant bay, and blue fountain bush and take as a drink with water.

Hernia

For the pain of a hernia, grind together a twig from a jackfruit tree, the roots of an elephant ear fig tree, and turpeth or St. Thomas lid pod. Chew the resulting mixture.

Menstrual Problems

For menstrual problems, grind to a fine powder 2.04117 grams of pepper, 2.04117 grams of black cumin, 4.08234 grams of long pepper, 16.3293 grams of drumstick tree leaves, 4.08234 grams of wild ginger, 4.08234 grams of sweet flag, and 4.08234 grams of small rhizome ginger. Dissolve in warm water and take as a drink.

For menstrual problems and haemorrhoids suffered by women, dry roast in a pan nutgall black seed, red entada bean (snuffbox sea bean), heart-leaved moonseed, grey nicker bean, chili, and five kinds of *umbelliferae* (fennel, anise or sweet fennel, cumin, black cumin, and dill). Remove from the pan and grind together to a fine powder. Dissolve in warm water and take as a drink.

Childbirth

For labour complications followed by a difficult delivery, take a square of red fabric and place it on the mother's abdomen above the baby's head in the fontanel area. This will enable an easier delivery.

Medicine for hypertension and haemorrhage during labour, take a sprig of a parasitic plant and grind with water to a pulpy consistency. Apply the ointment from head to toe. This will make delivery easier.

For easy childbirth, chant the following colloquial Pali mantra: *saw hti ka pa tha ingulimal ra tha*. While chanting the mantra, blow over a cup of water seven times. Pour on the head and belly button of the woman in labour.

Haemorrhoids (Dry Piles)

For haemorrhoids, grind together black cumin, opium, rosy leadwort, Himalayan gentian, roots of Indian ginseng or winter cherry, and pepper. Dissolve in water and take orally.

A second prescription for haemorrhoids, grind cowrie shell with the white seed of Indian wild liquorice and wild asparagus, and the peel of a ridge gourd. Dissolve in water in which rice has been soaked and drink.

A third prescription for haemorrhoids, grind together 7 ticals (114.3051 grams) of sweet flag, 5 ticals (81.6465 grams) of red physic nut or wild croton, 5 ticals (81.6465 grams) of tailed pepper, 4 ticals (65.3172 grams) of liquorice or sweet wood, 3 ticals (48.9879 grams) of rosy leadwort, 1 tical (16.3293 grams) of long pepper, and 2 ticals (32.6586 grams) of asafoetida. Dissolve in warm water and drink.

For haemorrhoids and inflammation of the stomach and small intestine, grind to a powder 8.16466 grams black cumin, 8.16466 grams of tamarind, 8.16466 grams of bark from the Indian gooseberry tree, 7 peppercorns, 7 long peppers, 8.16466 grams of dry roasted salt, and 3 pods of cardamom. Dissolve in warm water and drink.

Restoring Normal Body Function

Place in a pot of water the roots of a snowflake tree, roots of a blackboard tree or devil's tree, and 7 peppercorns. Bring to the boil over the fire and reduce the liquid from three parts water to one part water. Strain and take the liquid as a drink.

Mental Illness, Shock, Anxiety, and Insomnia

For loss of taste and symptoms of restlessness associated with an unstable mind, grind together 272.155 grams of long pepper, 272.155 grams of dog bush, 272.155 grams of nutmeg, 272.155 grams of asafoetida, 1,088.62 grams of golden shower, and 1,088.62 grams of pepper. Add water and take as a drink. This mixture can also be used as a massage lotion.

For anxiety leading to trembling and shaking with worry or causing body paralysis and pain, take Indian ipecac, roots of bitter cucumber, and black bat lily. Immerse in water drained from rice that has been soaked overnight. Strain the liquid and take as a drink.

For insomnia and a deranged mind, grind together rex begonia vine, chicken droppings, cat and dog excrement, human excrement, black cow urine, and 7 peppercorns. Rub the mixture onto the body.

For anxiety, eat a Java bean leaf with some green sugarcane juice.

For a feeling of uneasiness and disquiet, grind elephant ear leaves (night-scented lily), Indian ipecac, Indian bay seed, and millettia on a stone. Add water drained from rice that has been soaked overnight. Mix to a pulpy consistency. Take the mixture as a drink.

For mental instability caused by a shock, grind together to a fine powder nutmeg, cloves, five kinds of *umbelliferae* (fennel, anise or sweet fennel, cumin, black cumin, dill), pepper, black myrobalan, long pepper, liquorice or sweet wood, coriander seeds, and red sandalwood. Divide the powder into two parts. Use one part as an inhalant. Boil the other part with roots of bowing lady or tube flower. Strain and take as a drink.

Injuries Caused by Accidents

The text quotes as examples of accidents, falling from trees, and falling off the backs of cows and water buffaloes. Cut the roots, bark, and leaves from a blackboard tree or devil's tree and boil in water with some pepper. Take as a drink.

Low Disease Resistance

Fill a small cloth sack with herbal medicine (herbs not specified). Heat the sack by a fire. Apply to the body as a hot fomentation. Herbal bags can also be used for a medicinal bath treatment.

Fatigue

To relieve fatigue and feelings of weakness, take dog bush, shoots of elephant grass, young sugarcane, curry leaves, wild asparagus, onion, croton, and pepper. Immerse in water and bring to the boil. Strain and take as a drink. This potion can also be used as a herbal bath.

Restoring Normal Bodily Function

Take the roots of a snowflake tree, roots of a blackboard tree or devil's tree, and 7 peppercorns. Boil with three parts water and reduce to one part. Strain and take as a drink.

Insanity

For insanity and emotional hysteria, grind to a powder 5 ticals (81.6465 grams) each of 5 kinds of *umbelliferae* (fennel, anise or sweet fennel, cumin, black cumin, dill), 5 kinds of lily (white water lily, red water lily, blue lotus, pygmy water lily or small white water lily, and Indian lotus (sacred water lily), 1 tical (16.3293 grams) of fig tree root, 1 tical of Indian valerian, 1 tical of small rhizome ginger, 1 tical of scent gland from a musk deer, 1 tical Indian ipecac, 1 tical of rosy leadwort, 1 tical of Himalayan gentian, 1 tical of monkey pod tree (rain tree), 1 tical of cherimoya, 1 tical of yellow jade orchid tree, 1 tical of agarwood (eaglewood), 1 tical of bastard sandalwood, 1 tical of pepper, 1 tical of dog bush, 1 tical of Chinese finger ginger root, 1 tical of white or red sandalwood, 1 tical of rhino blood, 1 tical of sweet flag, and 1 tical of python's gall bladder. Grind the ingredients to a powder and mix with sugarcane, palm sugar, rock salt, and honey in a clean pot. Close the lid tightly and bury in amongst rice stored in the granary. Leave for seven days. Remove and take the mixture orally.

A body rub for someone who is insane, emotionally unstable, and hysterical, take hair from a widow who has had three husbands and grind with alum, green vitriol, borax, a sliver cut from the trunk of a fishtail palm, arsenic trisulphide, nutmeg, cloves, pepper, black turmeric, wild ginger, crude oil (kerosene), and dust from a termite hill. Measure the same amount of each ingredient and mix with pork fat until a pulpy consistency. Apply to the whole body. Take a laxative to achieve a bowel movement.

To cure a crazy or insane person, grind to a powder 5 *paan* leaves, asafoetida, nutmeg, cloves, willow-leaved justicia, Malabar nut, red castor bean, and 7 purging croton fruits. Weigh each ingredient to match the weight of the 5 *paan* leaves in the recipe. Take orally.

An inhalant for a crazy, insane, and hysterical person, take 7 young shoots of willow-leaved justicia, 7 young shoots from the potato tree or from velvet nightshade, black cumin, pepper, dwarf Indian olive, roots of cinnamon tree, thorn apple, or devil's trumpet, and peel from cardamom pods. Each ingredient should be the same weight. Grind together and wrap the mixture in a thin cotton cloth. Inhale three times every evening.

Paralysis

For treatment of paralysis, pound the shoots of elephant grass and black sacred garlic pear leaves together with a little white lime, quarried from limestone, and mix with water left over in a rice steaming pot. Place the pot in hot ash in the kitchen fire to heat up the mixture. Use a towel to absorb the warm mixture and wrap it around the hands and feet.

A second treatment for paralysis, grind together 4.08233 grams of nutmeg, 4.08233 grams of sweet flag, 8.18466 grams of cloves, [?] grams of long pepper, 2.04117 grams of green vitriol, 2.04117 grams of arsenic trisulphide, and 1.02058 grams of pepper. Take the resulting powder with water in which rice has been washed and fermented.

Mad Cow Disease

For fatal mad cow disease, grind together a bone from a black dog and a chameleon, a bone from a gibbon and a slow loris, a bone from a vulture, and the skull of a human struck by lightning. Add asafoetida, sesame, 10 measures of condensed milk, and earth from a field where sesame is grown. Recite the colloquial Pali mantra: *Kit sa aha mong mi awkar say tit hta.*

4. Controlling Evil Spirits, Ghosts, and Witches

Evil spirits are supernatural entities, harbingers of bad luck, sickness, and death. They can possess humans and animals. Ghosts are disembodied humans who because of evils committed in previous lives have been reborn to haunt the living. They are blamed for many forms of mental illness. Witches are malicious human beings who act out of hatred and spite either on their own volition or on behalf of clients. Their work is highly secretive. Witches are careful to hide their identity from those around them. Saya Sao

Silawan, one of the authors of this manuscript, was obviously familiar with witchcraft but we do not know from the text whether he was a practitioner himself.

Prescriptions used to control evil spirits contain ingredients that represent the beneficial power of Buddhism and the malignant power of evil. Combining good and evil involves using the power of beneficial spirits to heal a patient while controlling evil spirits to prevent their devious intervention. The healing power of Buddhism is transferred through Pali incantations and ingredients empowered by proximity to a sacred source, for example, mud collected from splatters on the hem of a monk's robe and fragments taken from a chipped alms bowl kept in the sanctity of a monastery ordination hall. The malignant power of evil spirits is controlled by profane ingredients like scrapings from human bone stolen from a cemetery and shavings from wooden poles used to turn corpses at cremation sites. Other ingredients include human and animal excrement, hair from suspect witches, polluted water, and disease-carrying insects. The act of stealing or secretly acquiring profane ingredients from cemeteries is repugnant and involves covert operations by practitioners of black magic.

Some ingredients are empowered by the force of nature, for example, shavings taken from the bark of trees struck by lightning and scrapings appropriated from the horns and skins of animals hit by lightning. A particularly potent ingredient is bone stolen from the corpse of a person who was killed in an act of human violence or who died in an accident or during a natural disaster. The spirit released suddenly from the deceased becomes a sadistic, wandering spirit out to cause mayhem, responsible for sickness and death in humans.

Practising black magic can be risky. Evil spirits are aggressive and difficult to control. They are the cause of chaos in society. They possess men who become drunk and disorderly, harass monks during Buddhist ceremonies, desecrate graves, and start vicious fights. Many become mentally unstable. These spirits can turn against *saya* trying to control them. If a *saya* loses control over evil spirits, he will try to exorcize them. He recites powerful Pali incantations praising the Attributes of the Buddha, the Eightfold Path, and the Triple Gem. He also uses prescriptions as given in this text. If these do not achieve the desired effect, he consults a devout monk whose source of power comes from self-discipline and strict observance of many Buddhist precepts. He may seek help from an experienced *saya* who observes Buddhist precepts and has greater power and knowledge of exorcism.

Powerful and aggressive prescriptions involving black magic are operated within a strict code. The potential victim must be an evil person who deserves to suffer. Permitted targets are those who cause serious physical and mental harm to others, and those who damage or destroy the property of others on at least three occasions. Those who live honest lives and observe at least five Buddhist precepts are not victimised. If black magic is aimed at an innocent person of high moral standing, that person will suffer no ill effects because their faith will protect them. However, this code operates according to the Buddhist lore of *karma*. Those who live blameless lives in this life cycle may be targeted if they committed serious offences in a previous life.

Counteracting Evil Spirits

This prescription counteracts witchcraft and acts carried out by evil human beings. It negates the malign power of sorcerers and ghosts. Scrape residue from a wooden cooking ladle used in the upper part of a rice steamer. Add shavings from a wooden house pillar, shavings from a wooden ladder leading to a monastery building, and from a wooden ladder leading up to a house. Also add shavings from the door of a house and from the door of a monastery. Grind together to a powder adding 7 rice grains collected from wastewater residue kept under the dish washing shelf and 7 green-headed flies.

Fever Caused by Evil Spirits

To counteract a fever and body aches caused by a spell cast by a witch, a sorcerer, or a ghost, wrap 816.465 milligrams of the powder from the recipe above for counteracting evil spirits with shavings taken from a banana tree trunk. Grill over a fire to expunge the spirits.

Counteracting Murder

To stop contract killers from murdering an individual. The contract killer is a witch, a human sorcerer, or an evil ghost. The intended victim must sit on a worn mat on the floor facing towards the east. He holds in his hands an old, chipped bowl made in the Shan State of Mong Kueng. The bowl is filled with powder (given in the previous prescription) for counteracting evil. The weight of the powder is matched to the number of contract assassins. Powder weighed to the equivalent of one seed of the rosary pea (272.155 milligrams) will kill one assassin. If the powder is weighed to the equivalent of two seeds of the rosary pea (544.210 milligrams), two contract killers will die. If the contents are weighed to the equivalent of three seeds of the rosary pea (816.365 milligrams), three will die.

Killing an Evil Spirit

To kill an evil spirit, ghost, or sorcerer. Grind together nutmeg, cloves, five kinds of *umbelliferae* (fennel, anise or sweet fennel, cumin, black cumin, dill), pepper, asafoetida, opium, wild ginger, sweet flag, and small rhizome ginger. Add 7 ground cockroaches, 7 shredded spiders' skins, 7 shredded horse fly skins, and 7 rice grains of leftover rice collected from a crack in a wooden mortar. Mix in 7 pieces of shaving taken from the outer strut of a wooden ladder, a hair from the head of 3 village headmen, a hair from the head of 3 widows, and shaving from the bone of a human corpse. Collect a little black charcoal residue from a cremation site, shavings from a wooden pole used to turn burning corpses during cremation, soil from a graveyard, and alfalfa grass growing by a graveyard. Add 33 scrapings of tree root growing across a path, 33 scrapings from a tree stump by a path, thousands of different flowers [*sic*], 33 shoots from different trees, 33 pieces of plant root growing in water, and wood from 3 trees that have been struck by lightning. This powerful recipe can only be prepared on the auspicious days Tuesday and Saturday. During preparation, a *sutta* is chanted seven times to ward off evil spirits.

Possession

To cure a person who is possessed by a witch or an evil sorcerer. Grind to a powder the shavings of burnt wood from a funeral pyre, sweet flag, thorn apple, Indian ivy rue, pepper, and dog bush. Take orally with water or use as a body rub or massage lotion.

Hungry Ghosts and Spirits

A cure for a person demonically possessed by an evil spirit with an enormous appetite. Grind together 7 shredded bed bug skins, 7 shredded spider skins, earth taken from 7 steps of a house ladder, and 3 pieces of stick lac stuck on wood or bamboo under the roof of a house. Take orally with warm water.

To drive away witches, evil sorcerers, and spirits with enormous appetites. Grind together 1,088.62 milligrams of arsenic trisulphide, 1,088.62 milligrams of Ridley's staghorn fern, and 4 seeds of white rosary pea or seeds of Indian wild liquorice. Apply as a body rub.

To treat a person captured by or under the spell of ghosts, evil spirits with enormous appetites, demons, or witches. This recipe can also be used to treat someone possessed by spirits craving human meat and bones, and a person who accidently collides with an unknown spirit. Grind together black leadwort, rosy leadwort, white leadwort, Ceylon oak, blackberry lily or candy lily, pepper, money plant or devil's ivy, giant fern tree, cardamom, and sweet flag. Add ground bone from a human killed by lightning, wood from a tree struck by lightning, and extract from a tiger's head. Mix in ground bone and horn from a white buffalo struck by lightning, ground bone from a human who died in violent circumstances, ground bone of a python, skin shed by a snake, ground bone from a black dog, a black chicken, a black cat, and a black crow. Add sand collected from the middle of a path, a hornet taken from a hornet's nest by a graveyard, and a piece of crushed tile taken from the floor close to a Buddha image. Add earth from a pigsty, mud from the hem of a monk's robe, mud from a door, and mud from a baby's shirt. Mix with 7 rice grains taken from the bottom of a mortar, 7 cracked rice grains, 7 shredded spider skins, 7 thin bamboo strips, the tail of a long-tailed king crow, and the tail of a falcon. Add mud from a nest of the mud dauber wasp, chippings from a cracked pot used at the shrine to the guardian spirit of a town, and a piece from the crack in an alms bowl used inside the ordination hall of a Buddhist monastery. Add a dung beetle, green flies, a centipede, a bumblebee, a cockroach, and a few winged termites. Grind all the dead and living ingredients together to a powder and place in a bamboo basket. Leave in a place recommended by the *saya*. Chant a *sutta* for three nights to ward off further harm to the victim.

Cannibal Spirits

A cure to drive away spirits craving human meat and bones. Grind together a stick of firewood, a piece of wood from a tree struck by lightning, earth from a graveyard, human ashes from a graveyard, rabbit droppings, wild ginger, yellow turmeric, white turmeric root, asafoetida, and water pepper. Take the powder orally with warm water.

An Injection for a Bewitched Person

Grind together 7 white seeds of Indian or Jamaican wild liquorice, 7 long pepper corns, 7 regular pepper corns, 7 slices of wild ginger, 7 slices of small turmeric, 7 slices of small rhizome ginger, shavings from the trunk of fishtail palm, 1.02058 grams of yellow cinnabar, and 7 slices of sweet flag. Strain, mix with lime sap, and inject under the skin.

Folios 5–8

Folios 9–12

31

Folios 13–16

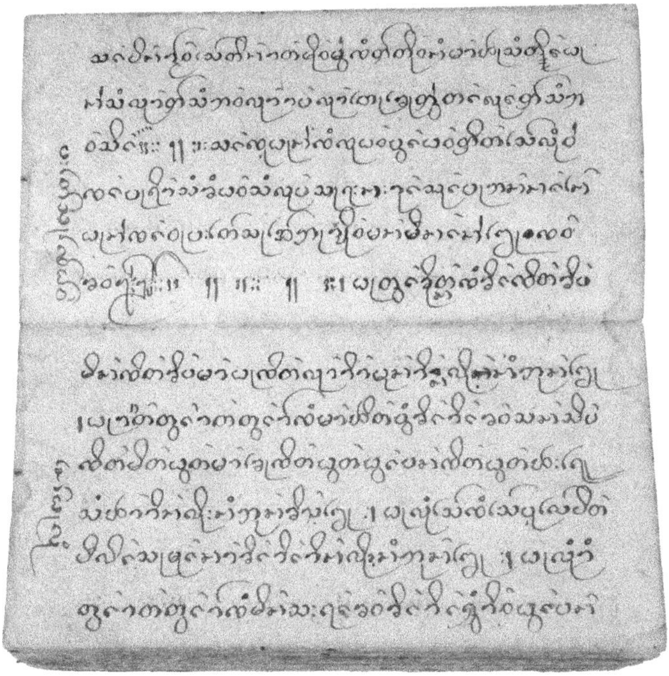

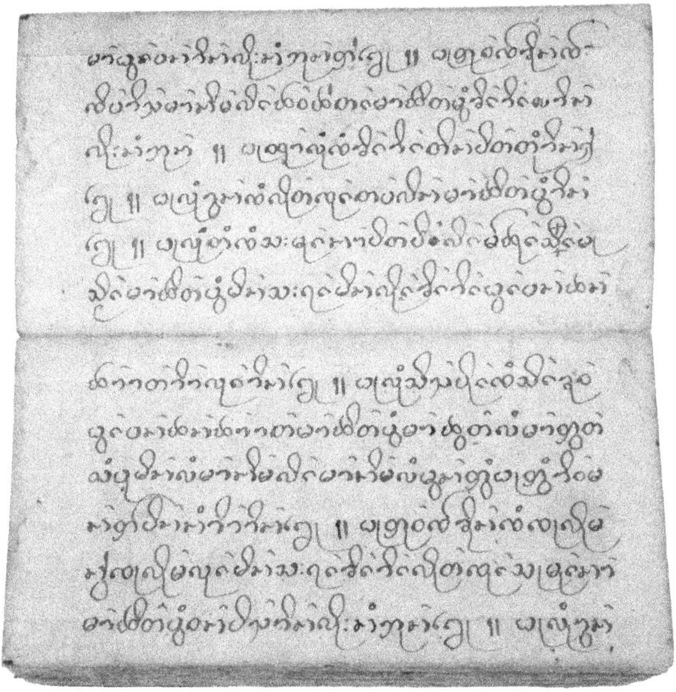

Folios 17–20

Folios 21–24

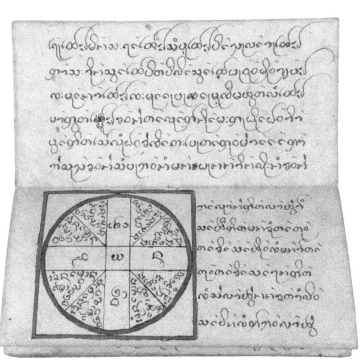

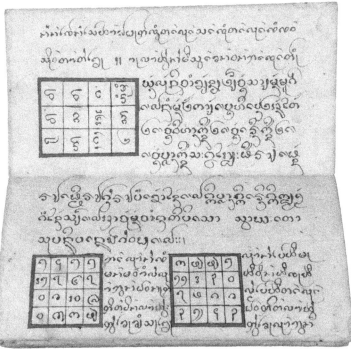

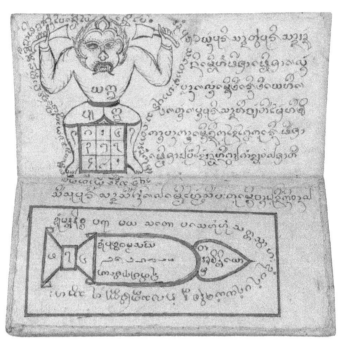

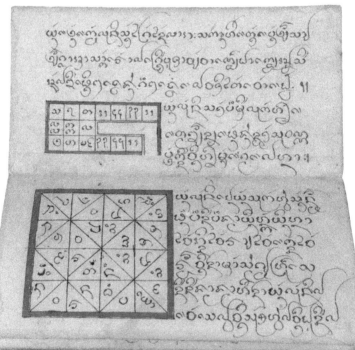

Folios 151–154

36

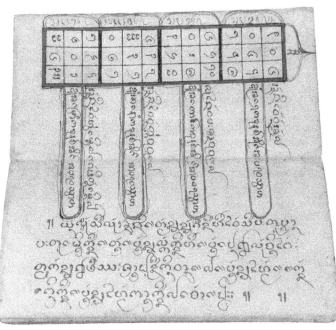

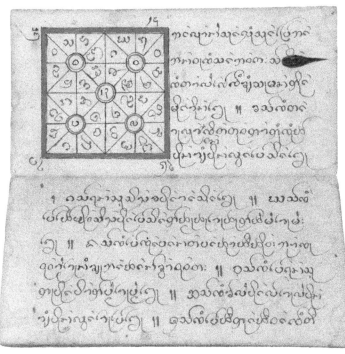

Folios 155–158

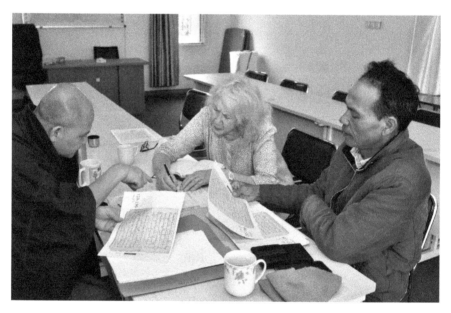

Phra Viccita, Abbot of Shan State Buddhist University, with Zaray Saw (Sai Seng), an expert on Shan manuscripts, and the author Susan Conway examining a copy of the Horniman manuscript, Shan State Buddhist University, 2019.

Chapter 2

MYSTICAL DIAGRAMS (*YANTRA*)

Yantra are mystical diagrams containing abbreviations for Pali incantations and *katha* (magic spells). They also contain numbers representing the life force of planets, prime numbers, which are considered innately powerful, and instructional symbols. The Horniman manuscript has ten folios of *yantra* and two folios of drawings. *Yantra* function as a form of protection and as mechanisms for healing. Letters, syllables, and phrases are placed in coded grid systems created by monks and *saya* (experts in the arts of the supernatural). For example, the syllable *o* is used as shorthand for *om*, in turn shorthand for the Pali incantation *om mani padme hum*, the mantra of Avalokiteshvara, the bodhisattva of compassion. Syllables of a secular nature include *na*, *ma*, *ba*, *ka*, and *da*, representing the elements water, air, earth, fire, and wind that are balanced in a healthy body but imbalanced in people who are sick. Symbols can represent instructions to a *saya* for breathing and blowing on clients during healing and cleansing rituals. Or they signify noises communicated by spirits and the utterances of humans who are possessed.

Pali incantations and *katha* appear together in *yantra*. Both are chanted in certain ceremonies. The Thai anthropologist Kraisri Nimmanahaeminda noted that in Northern Thai rituals, *yantra* displayed on banners contained Pali phrases and *katha*. During a protection ceremony held in Chiang Mai, he noted that a monk chanted in Pali to appeal to the Buddha to protect the city of Chiang Mai against uncontrolled spirits.[1] Then a *saya* chanted a *katha* in the local language that appealed to protective spirits not to cause harm to the city.[2] *Yantra* are used on a more permanent basis to protect buildings, villages, and cities. They are incised in wood, brick, and metal and inserted in walls and in lintels over doorways. A *saya* charges the protective power of *yantra*, appealing to the spirits and to local gods and goddesses, particularly Mae Kala who lives in the heavens and oversees affairs on earth, and Nang Sulat Suwalee who protects Buddhist scriptures. Their power is particularly strong on Wednesdays and Fridays in November (the 12th month of the Shan calendar), and on Saturdays and Buddhist holy days in March (the 4th month of the Shan calendar).

1. Kraisri Nimmaenhaeminda, 'The Lawa Guardian Spirits of Chiangmai', *Journal of the Siam Society*, 1967, 55 (BE 2527): 185–225.

2. Amphay Doré, *L'école de la Forêt: un itinéraire spirituel lao*, Aurangabad, India: Kailash Books, 1992, pp. 249–53.

1. Folio 148

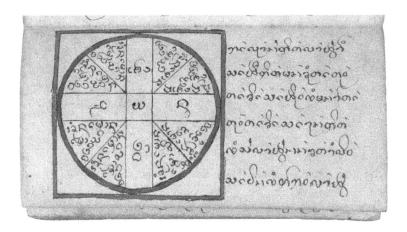

This circular *yantra* is for protection. It is known as the 'Five Buddha' *yantra*. The four past Buddhas and the Buddha of the future are represented in letters in the central cross. It is inscribed on small strips of metal kept in a leather pouch attached to a chain and worn as a bracelet on the wrist or upper arm, or as a necklace.

2. Folio 149

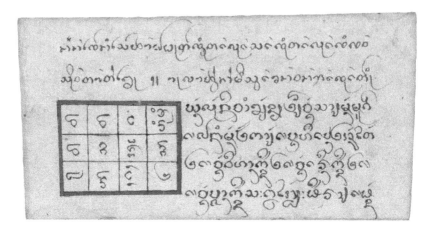

This *yantra* protects against evil spirits entering a home. It is copied on mulberry paper, rolled up and bound with cotton thread to a candle wick and inserted in a hollow beeswax candle. The candle is lit by a *saya* who offers incantations while walking and tipping the candle so that the wax drips on the floor to mark the outline of a sacred space that evil spirits cannot enter. In an alternative ritual, the *yantra* is copied on four separate sheets of mulberry paper. Each sheet is rolled up and bound with cotton to a candle wick and immersed in four separate bowls of oil. One bowl is placed in each of the cardinal directions.[3] Incantations to banish evil spirits are chanted while the wicks burn. This *yantra* can also protect children against nightmares. It is copied on cotton cloth and placed under the child's pillow or incised in silver and worn by the child as a necklace.

---

3. Interview with the Venerable Sai Khemacari, Wat Chieng Yin, Keng Tung, 2011.

3. Folio 150

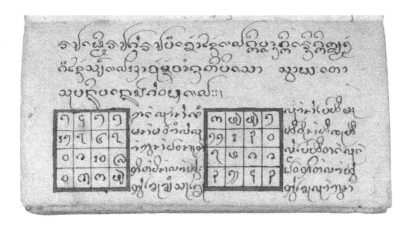

These *yantra* draw on the power of the planets, natural forces, and the god Indra. The *yantra* on the left has sixteen squares. The top row contains numerals 5, 4, 5, and 5 to make a total of 19 that represents the power of the planet Jupiter. In the second row, the first square contains the number 15 representing the power of the moon, followed by 7, an indivisible magic number, then 6 to signify the power of the sun, then a repeat of the number 7. In the third row, *o* represents the Pali phrase *om mani padme hum* followed by the letter *n*, followed by 10 to represent the power of Saturn, followed by an unrecognised symbol. In the fourth row, *ba* represents the power of earth, *ka* is for fire, *ka* is repeated, then the syllable *phya* represents the god Indra. The *yantra* on the right-hand side, top row, has the phrases *ka* for fire, *phya* and *phya*, repeated for Indra, and the number 5. The second row contains 11, an indivisible number, followed by a mystery symbol, then 3 and *o* for the Pali phrase *om mani padme hum*. The third row contains 7, then *pa* for the power of natural forces, *ka*, and *ka* for fire. In the fourth row, 3 is followed by an unidentified symbol, then 4 and 3.

These *yantra* resist all types of danger and prevent malignant spirits, ghosts, and witches from haunting villages, private dwellings, and monasteries. Each *yantra* is copied on five separate sheets of mulberry paper.

A length of candle wick is cut into five pieces weighing 2.04117 grams each. Sesame oil is weighed into five amounts of 81.6465 grams and poured into the lamps. The wick and *yantra* are placed in the oil. The lamps are lit and placed in five directions on the boundary of the area to be protected. The colloquial Pali mantra *ithipiso swakhataw supatipanaw* is chanted three, or up to seven times while the lamps are burning.

4. Folio 151

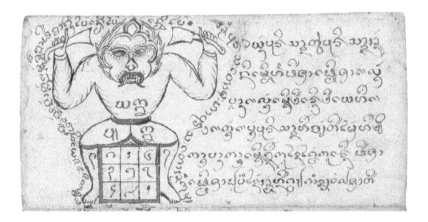

This freehand drawing depicts the ogre *phi lo*, a powerful spirit ogre, popular in Shan State. His image is copied on mulberry paper and incised in metal for protection. On a larger scale, the image is carved in wood and cut in brick to protect buildings. It is also stamped on cakes of soap (*sompoy*) distilled from acacia (*Acacia rugata Mer*) used in purification rituals.

Phi lo has the power to drive away spirits that place obstacles in the way of ambitious people and banish evil spirits causing illness. *Phi lo* is a frightening creature with no neck, an accepted characteristic of lower beings. He has red eyes, prominent teeth, and curled fangs protruding from exaggerated hairy lips. His chest is broad and tapers to a narrow-belted waist above a short loincloth. He wears a crown of flames. The word *yakka* (spirit) is written on his chest. He brandishes knives that resemble meat cleavers, symbols of cannibalism. Balanced between his thighs is a magic nine-square *yantra* containing numbers that add up to 15 when counted vertically, diagonally, and horizontally. The number 15 represents the power of the moon.[4] A Pali

---

4. In Shan astrology, the seven days of the week are reconfigured to eight time periods by splitting Wednesday into a before noon period and an after noon period. The eight are matched to the Sun, Moon, Mars, Mercury, Jupiter, Venus, Saturn, and Rahu (demon god of the moon who causes eclipses). Each planet is allocated a 'life force'.

text encircles the figure of *phi lo*, intended as a restraint on his power. If uncontrolled, *phi lo* becomes a destructive spirit.

In a ritual held in Shan State, images of *phi lo* are carved in wood or drawn on banners and paraded to appease guardian spirits. When the ritual is held in a town, the image is carried to the shrine of the town guardian spirit. If in a village, it is taken in procession to the main village shrine and, if for the protection of an individual house, carried to the spirit shrine in the garden. The colloquial Pali incantation *om puri tha taw maha puri tha taw* is chanted during the ritual.

5. Folio 152

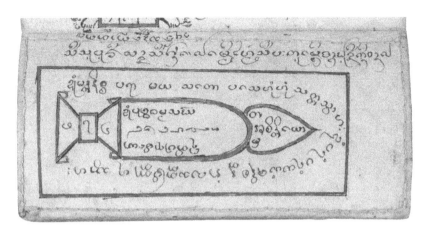

This depiction of a candle on a stand follows directly on the next folio after the image of *phi lo*. The candle is surrounded by written instructions for a candle ritual to exorcise evil spirits that cause illness. The image of *phi lo* from the previous folio is copied on a small sheet of mulberry paper and the name of the sick person, and the day, time, and year of the person's birth, are added. The paper is rolled up with a fragment of clothing belonging to the person and bound together with a candle wick using white cotton thread. A photograph of the sick person may be substituted for the fragment of clothing. The bundle is rolled in softened beeswax to create a candle. The candle is lit at a time specified by a *saya*, calculated according to the birth data of the ill person. While the candle burns, the incantation *ang hae kwang* and good luck incantation *thien suk lap luk wan* are chanted and the power of *phi lo* is invoked to drive away evil spirits. The colloquial Pali incantation *om puri tha taw maha puri tha taw* is also chanted during the ritual.

6. Folio 153

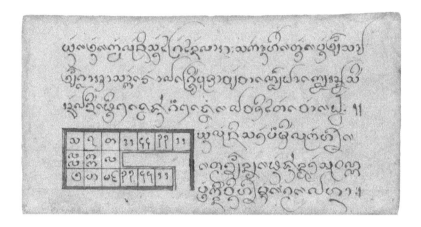

Yantra are formulated specifically with spaces left vacant. In this rectangular *yantra*, the space is a gap of five squares representing a void in space (*pong pheuw*) that draws suffering and unhappiness into it.[5] It is prescribed to childless couples. Incised on a small silver or gold plate, it is attached to a chain and worn by the childless woman as a necklace or bracelet. The *yantra* is also copied on mulberry paper, bound up with a candle wick, and inserted in a hollow wax candle. The couple light the candle and offer a set of incantations while the candle burns.

5. Interview with the monks of Wat Chieng Yin, Keng Tung, 2011.

7. Folio 154

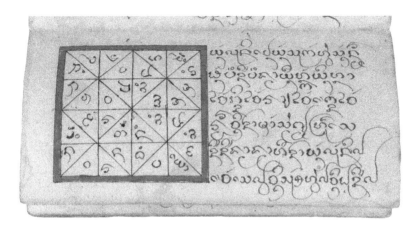

This *yantra* is used in rituals to promote good luck. An offering tray to appease the spirits is prepared in advance. Offerings placed on the tray include a triangular paper pennant, 6 ticals of dried tea leaves (6 ticals = 97.9758 grams), 4 chunks of sugarcane, and 5 lumps of beeswax.

There are three methods for conducting the ritual. For the first, the *yantra* is copied on mulberry paper and burnt in a dish of oil while incantations are offered. For the second, the *yantra* is etched on the surface of one or up to three beeswax candles with the birth date of the client etched below the *yantra*. The candles are lit, and incantations offered. For the third method, the birth data and the name of the client are written on mulberry paper rolled up, bound with a cotton candle wick, and inserted in a hollow beeswax candle. Incantations are offered while the candle burns.

This *yantra* can be a means to treat mental stress, nightmares, and sleeplessness, and can also cure breathlessness. It is copied on mulberry paper and soaked in water that contains dissolved soap pods (*Senegalia rugata*). The soapy water is charged by the power of the *yantra*. The *yantra* is removed from the soapy water that is used as a shampoo. Alternately, the *yantra* can be immersed in scented water for a set amount of time. The *yantra* is removed and the water poured slowly over the head of the patient.

8. Folio 155–156

This *yantra* is spread across two folios. At the top are four squares with faded pencil numbers 1–7 written above them. The four squares below are divided into nine equal-sized squares containing auspicious numbers ranging from 0 to 311. Four ribbon-shaped strips below the squares represent the cardinal directions. A set of instructions is given for each strip. Reading from left to right:

1. Place this *yantra* to the eastern side.

Incantations: *aha pa ya wa thwar ha* and 'Om, seven pools of water on the eastern side'

2. Place this yantra to the southern side.

Incantations: *aha pa ya wa thwar ha* and 'Om, seven pools of water on the southern side'

3. Place this yantra to the western side.

Incantations: *aha pa ya wa thwar ha* and 'Om, seven pools of water on the western side'

4. Place this yantra to the northern side.

Incantations: *aha pa ya wa thwar ha* and 'Om, seven pools of water on the northern side'.[6]

In the past, attacks on Shan regional cities and states were part of local power struggles between courts. Principalities rose, flourished, and declined, constantly subject to attack from neighbouring states and foreign powers. Some were devastated by disease outbreaks and famines that killed thousands. The Shan fortified their cities with moats, walls, and gates that locked at night. They called on guardian spirits for protection. This *yantra* helps protect against enemy invasion and defeat in battle. It could also be charged to prevent disease epidemics and famine. The *yantra* was etched on metal, brick, or wood in sets of four pieces. One piece was placed in each of the four cardinal directions, usually inserted in a boundary wall or in a plinth above town gates. If wood was used, the preferred choice was scented hardwood, naturally dried. When there was a disease outbreak, or famine was predicted, eight *yantra* were inserted in gates and walls in the cardinal and sub-cardinal directions to reinforce protection. When there was damage and walls needed to be rebuilt, damaged *yantra* were replaced and rededicated.[7]

---

6. The phrase 'pools of water' may refer to moats outside city walls, built as part of defences, or to the direction of wells.

7. The monks of Wat Jong Kham, Keng Tung, provided this information, 2011.

9. Folio 157

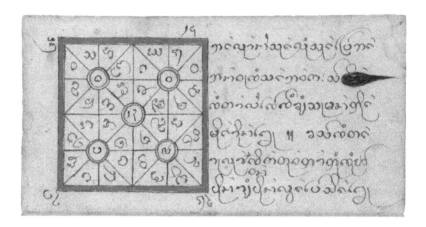

This *yantra* can be adapted to suit individual needs. Thirty-two letters drawn inside triangles are contained in four squares. Five circles contain letters that can be altered, for example, to cure a named disease instead of a non-specific illness. The text states this *yantra* can only be used to create positive power, in other words, to heal.

10. Folio 163

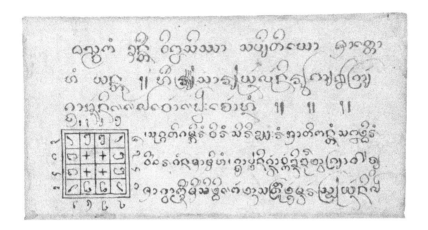

This square *yantra* is divided into sixteen small squares with letters and symbols inside and outside the square. Offering protection against all forms of danger, it is copied on mulberry paper, folded up small, and given to the client to swallow. The following incantation in colloquial Pali is chanted to invoke the power of protective spirits: *Namaw damatha razataw pannateda etamay gilarni yanihta wiyupakkha udaetar ahpaytar dissakan khanti wipathitha sabitiyaw ahat htaw hanyantu.*

11. Folio 164

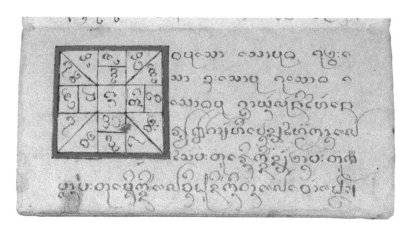

This *yantra* has a central cross divided into nine squares. The surrounding four squares contain eight triangles. Letters and syllables are shorthand for Pali incantations.[8] This *yantra* creates a healthy state of mind and the ability to speak well in public. It is copied on mulberry paper, rolled up and bound together with a cotton wick, and immersed in a shallow dish of vegetable oil. The wick is lit, and incantations are offered to invoke the power of the goddess Nang Sulat Siwalee, protector of Buddhist scriptures and guardian of actors, performers, and public speakers.[9] When the wick burns out, residual ash is collected and diluted in coconut milk. Droplets of sap collected from a freshly cut branch of a ficus tree, honey gathered from wild bees, and sugarcane juice are added. This concoction of fruit and magical power guarantees a gentle, confident, and persuasive voice. Mantra: *Daputhaw thawpuda buddathaw ahthawpu buthawda thawdapu.*

An alternative prescription involves preparing the drink as above but excluding the ash. It is poured into a dish and a copy of the *yantra* drawn

8. A monk from Wat Chieng Yin, Keng Tung, described this as 'incorrectly spelled Pali'.

9. According to legend, Nang Sulat Siwalee protected the Buddha against Manee Mae Kala, goddess of death, who competed with the Buddha in a struggle for power.

on mulberry paper is immersed for a prescribed time to allow its power to be absorbed.[10] The *yantra* is removed and the reinforced drink is consumed. Auspicious days for this ritual are Wednesdays and Fridays in November (the 12th month of the Shan lunar calendar), or Saturdays and Buddhist holy days in March (the 4th month of the Shan lunar calendar). Other auspicious times may be calculated by a *saya* who consults astrological charts.

This *yantra* can be used as a form of protection when inscribed on wood and secured at the entrance to a property. If a house, the *yantra* is nailed on the entrance door; if a village, over the entrance arch; and if a town or city, four copies are placed over the entrance gates.[11] The incantation offered at the time of instigation is *Sugato gambhiram wiram sirigaram ahtikantan thabadiram weetayagan namarmihan.*

When this incantation is chanted backwards it gives defenders the skill, competence, and fearlessness to conquer enemies.

---

10. A saya admitted that this prescription is not as powerful as when ash is included.

11. At the time the Horniman manuscript was written in the early nineteenth century, skirmishes between rival Tai groups required villages and towns to be protected both physically and spiritually.

Conclusion

Certain herbs have been in use for healing and ritual for thousands of years. Seven thousand years ago, ginger was an ingredient used in Austronesian remedies. It had ritual significance in appeasing the spirits to protect sailors and seafaring canoes. Many plant ingredients listed in these prescriptions have a long history of medicinal and ritual use. However, in the time since this manuscript was written, tropical forests and local habitats where a huge variety of plants were abundant have been destroyed by intensive farming, logging, mineral extraction, and indiscriminate housing development. Prescriptions like the one in the Horniman manuscript that requires fifty plant ingredients are a thing of the past. Although the prescriptions recorded here may be redundant, that does not mean they have no value in today's world. The manuscript is a wealth of information for conservationists who can compare the list of flora and fauna available to healers in the past with what is available today in depleted forests.

Among the ingredients listed in the manuscript are plants and herbs grown in home gardens, usually tended by women who cultivated fruit vegetables and herbs for medicinal use. Today, working practices and pressure on land means there are fewer home gardens. Some women herbalists in Shan State still grow their own, and there are monasteries where monks cultivate herbs that they use to make pills with a limited range of ingredients. It is a long way from the world of the missionary Leslie Milne, quoted earlier, who noted that knowledge and use of herbs was widespread. Such skills are not widely shared today. Who would concoct such complicated therapies when a visit to a local pharmacy provides an instant herbal preparation over the counter?

This manuscript contains ingredients extracted from wild animals trapped in the forest. Culling bears, tigers, pangolins, rhinoceroses, and snakes to extract ingredients for medicines is now illegal. Legislation is vital to protect what is left of a dwindling population. Conditions were different in the nineteenth century. Wild animals were abundant. Many foreign travellers in the nineteenth century described their fear of attack in Shan forests. They slept in trees to escape tigers that were prolific. The possibility of being mauled was taken seriously. This manuscript contains a prescription for ointment to treat torn flesh caused by tiger claws and a *katha* chanted to protect against attack. Tigers were hunted for their bones, which was ground in medicine, and for their hair, whiskers, and teeth that were made into protective talismans. It is estimated today there are only twenty-two wild tigers remaining in the whole of Myanmar. In eastern Shan State, a temple was recently built in their memory after what was thought to be the last remaining tiger killed in the hills. An elderly man told me that when he was a child the distant roar of a tiger was a common sound. Rhinoceroses were hunted in local forests for their horn that was ground in medicines. Small populations may exist in remote areas of Myanmar but not in Shan State. Bears were prolific, and up to fifty years ago local people reported lethal attacks. Bears were hunted for bile used to treat a range of ailments. The Myanmar sun bear is now on the vulnerable list of the International Union of Conservation of Nature (IUCN). Pangolins were hunted for their scales. Today, they are the most trafficked animals, sent to China and Vietnam, an illegal trade that continues to flourish. Pythons were hunted for their bile. Today, the python is listed as vulnerable on the IUCN red list but there is no record of numbers remaining in Shan state.

When Western-trained physicians began to practise in Shan State, their approach to medicine was very different from local practitioners. Western-trained doctors challenged the lack of uniformity in diagnostic techniques and treatments in traditional medicine. They wanted standardisation and the study of Western medical textbooks to be the norm. Manuscripts, recognised as containers of traditional knowledge, coexisted with Western textbooks until the 1950s. Respect for local belief systems in treating patients dwindled although practice continued, particularly in rural areas. Today, some people take both forms of treatment. Herbalists treat patients also receiving care from Western-trained doctors. For example, a patient with

HIV attends a government clinic where he receives the latest drugs. He also goes to a herbalist who treats the cough and skin infections associated with HIV. Western medicine and herbal remedies deal with physical illness, and the Shan keep faith in the psychological value of prayer, meditation, and ritual. Those defining the rituals associated with treating sickness emphasise the contribution of monks and *saya* today. They speak of an ability to 'extend life force, float away evil from the body, mind, and spirit, bring good luck, and dispense *metta*', Pali for loving-kindness, benevolence, and harmony.

The Horniman manuscript is an historic record of treatments to cure mind and body. As repositories of knowledge, old manuscripts act as references for monks and *saya* practising today. They modify and adapt prescriptions to suit modern ways of life and to meet current political and economic circumstances. Shan refugees have fled to Thailand to escape war and poverty in Shan State. Many are destitute squatters. Without formal registration in Thailand, they have no employment rights or access to health care. They flock to monasteries in a state of anxiety hoping for assistance. Traditional healing is provided by Shan monks and *saya* living in exile. Time taken to listen and be sympathetic to their plight is a calming process supported by healing rituals. There is a charge for treatment, but monks often waive fees telling patients to return when they have found a job and earned some money.

Pressure of numbers seeking help means the production of ritual materials, particularly *yantra*, is often speeded up with the use of photocopiers and pre-packaged materials. An example of this is seen in the historic candle ritual, recorded in this manuscript in the *yantra* section. A modern method involves wrapping together in cellophane hollow wax candles, candle wicks, and *yantra* on mulberry paper with an appropriate incantation included. Several different packages are produced. A label attached to the cellophane tells which illness or period of bad luck a particular package treats. The client pays a fee for the package, assembles the candle, and performs the ritual in the monastery or at home. When the candle stops burning, the ash residue is saved and diluted in blessed water provided by the monastery. It is taken as a curative drink, or the ash is mixed with oil and smeared on the body as a form of protection.

In another adaptation of the candle ritual, a monk has created a set of healing *yantra* based on a fusion of Shan, Thai, and Burmese *yantra*. He has tested them through trial and error. If patients report one is particularly effective, it becomes part of regular use. If ineffective, the monk adjusts the *yantra* and tries again. If it still does not work, he discards it. The sheer volume of requests has led him to streamline the system with the assistance of novice monks. The set of *yantra* he dispenses regularly are taken to a printing shop close to the monastery where photocopies are made. Novices go there regularly to top up supplies for the abbot to prescribe. He keeps them close to hand in a drawer in his consulting room. They treat a range of conditions. Not all are for sickness. Some are prescribed for good luck. Businessmen and local officials go to ask for success at work. The abbot describes the letters and symbols in the *yantra* he creates as *kha-tha thon-pis*, 'sacred words to withdraw negative power'.

Among settled communities, there are requests for protective rituals to bless motorcycles and cars. *Yantra* are attached to the windscreen of vehicles and to the handlebars of motorcycles. Vehicles are blessed with holy water and incantations are offered for protection from the cardinal directions, a change from previous centuries when spatial protection was sought against war, famine, and disease.

During the past few years, manuscripts written on *saa* paper have been catalogued and digitised along with manuscripts on palm leaf and other organic materials. Digital libraries with manuscripts in their collections now exist in Thailand, Laos, the United Kingdom, the United States, Germany, and Ireland. Anyone from anywhere in the world can search and view the images but there is little information on content. When content is added to the data base, it is likely that Buddhist texts will take preference. This is an important issue, as in terms of genre Shan medical treatises should be prioritised as they make up only a small percentage of overall subject matter. Fortunately, the Horniman manuscript is kept in excellent condition in a museum store with the writing clearly legible. It is not known how many similar texts are in good condition. At Shan State Buddhist University, a digital library is in the process of being created. It is hoped research will cover a wide range of topics. Students at the university who have graduated with an MA in Shan material culture and anthropology, have conducted fieldwork on manuscript cultures in rural monasteries. They have shown interest in the history and practice of traditional medicine and share digital images of *yantra* and esoteric material. Several chose this subject for their dissertations.

This book would be incomplete without refence to the character and quality of the script in the Horniman manuscript, written in a unique style distinct from Thai and Burmese script. Local writing materials are used. Black ink is made from soot mixed with animal or fish bile, or sap from the wild plant *ya muk* used as a binder. Making ink from natural ingredients is considered superior to Chinese block ink sold in local markets. Red dye is used to draw outlines of the *yantra* and to mark the end of passages in the text. It is made from lac, the resinous secretion of the lac insect. The handwriting flows evenly across the page. Letters have swirling tails, finished with a flourish. These visual characteristics give the Horniman manuscript an artistic value that complements the important information it contains.

Chapter 3

MAGIC SPELLS (*KATHA*)

This list of magic spells (*katha*) from the Horniman manuscript was provided by Saya Long Te Za and Saya Long Noi Na. The translation of symptoms into English was provided by Khun Tun Yee. They can be matched to symptoms described in the main text. At the end of this list are three prescriptions for success. They involve drinking water empowered by a *yantra* or using it as a face wash. *Katha* written on these *yantra* are not specified.

Katha Kya Ju Tham Pian. For general protection against evil.

Katha Hya Kae Laed. To cure headaches and stomach disorders.

Katha Hya Tha Pang. To cure painful eye infections that cause redness and swelling.

Katha Thum Khong Pi Pur Pi Sur (Hsa Pur). To exorcise ghosts that haunt the body and take control of the mind.

Katha Hya Ar Thad. To neutralise the harmful power of a potion administered by an inexperienced *saya*, for example, medicine that contains an ingredient of ash collected after burning an incorrectly written *yantra*, or a piece of fabric printed with an incorrect *yantra* that was swallowed.

Katha Hya Thuk Mai Thuk Tham. To cure a fever and restore normal temperature to a person who is cold.

Katha Hya Khya. To provide a general cure for those in a poor state of health.

Katha Hya Sae Yo. To cure stomach problems.

Katha Hya Ai/Hsa Loam. To treat a persistent cough and sore throat.

Katha Mat Hsur. To provide protection against attack by wild animals in the jungle.

Katha Hya Tong Jiep. To cure illnesses of the digestive tract.

Ka Ta Ang Hae Kwang and *Ka Ta Thien Suk Lap Luk Wan*. It is not clear from the text what these *katha* treat.

Katha Hya Tha Wod Jiep. To cure painful eye ailments and blindness caused by lack of treatment.

Katha Nae Hya Lerd Haeng. To cure blood clots and to stop haemorrhaging.

Katha Kon Kwang Lerd Yong Lerd Wa. This *katha* is part of the cure for mental disorders or insanity (translated as 'mad and crazy').

Katha Kon Yo Lerd Yu. To cure people who are anaemic and have a skin disease.

Katha Hya Ngan. To treat the body in a state of shock resulting from a fever or chills.

Katha Hya Khaeng Dai Pak. To cure paralysis of the body and bring feeling back to limbs.

Katha Hya Loam Lu (*Loam Kheun*). To cure general ill health, high blood pressure, and painful skin lesions.

Katha Pong Hsam Tha. To help remember events from the past and predict the future.

Katha Hya Khya Na. To cure skin abnormalities and infections on the face and body.

Katha Hya Kae Nao. This *katha* is a general cure for illness.

Katha Muk Ka La Long. To plan the future to ensure success in life.

Katha Tham Pian. To protect a person troubled by ghosts and evil spirits that appear in dreams. The person fears the apparitions will come alive to haunt them.

Katha Hya Long Hsa Kyam. This *katha* has all-encompassing power to cure evil.

Katha Hya Pi Pur (*Teuk Pur*). To protect the body and mind against evil ghosts and spirits that try to take control.

Katha Teuk Pi. To resist the power of ghosts and evil spirits.

Katha Hya Ma Hyo. To treat women who suffer menstrual pain and haemorrhage.

Katha Nae Hya Tham. To help cure painful flesh wounds caused by a cut from a sharp instrument.

Katha Hya Theuk Ka La. To cure people with undiagnosed symptoms.

Katha Hya Tha Jiep. To cure painful red eyes.

Katha Hya Lerd Lu. To cure dry skin and blood loss.

Katha Hya Tha Pae Tha Mo. To cure tired, itchy eyes.

Katha Hya Nuk Khong. To treat a seriously ill patient who is close to death.

Katha Hya Ho Khai. To cure headaches and dizziness.

Katha Hya Tha Pae Tha Pang. To cure eye diseases and blindness.

Ka Ta Sya Kae Na. To protect travellers wherever they go.

Katha Nae Hya Song Hon. To cure vomiting and illnesses of the digestive tract.

Katha Hya Tha Pae. To cure eye complaints.

There are some *katha* in the Horniman manuscript where the actual words are not written down. The text says a *katha* [no detail] is combined with *ma ha ni yom* magic, written on mulberry paper, and soaked in water for a specific time. The mulberry paper is removed from the water then used to cleanse the face. It helps prove innocence and prevent conviction in a court case. Using the same method, another *katha* brings success in road building, but in this prescription the builder must drink the magic water, not use it to wash his face. To improve intellect and bring success in life, again the water is taken as a drink.

Folios 25–28

Glossary

betel (*piper betle*): a leaf chewed with other ingredients, including areca palm nut (*areca catechu*), tobacco, and white lime

candle ritual: a candle made from hot wax rolled around a wick bound with a *yantra* written on paper or cloth

Chula Sakarat: a lunisolar calendar

cinnabar: mercuric sulphide

dua tham: a general term for Lan Na, Tai Khoen, and Tai Lue scripts

dukka (Pali): suffering and its causes

eight time periods: a Tai counting system used in divination

ekeavisati: a tiger spirit

gatha/katha: numbers, letters, and symbols read as magical incantations

gradaat saa: mulberry paper used for manuscripts

karma (*kam*): the law of cause and effect

katha: a magic spell

khan kru: an altar

lacquer: made from the resin of the tree *gluta usitata*

leporello: a manuscript that folds in one continuous sheet like a concertina

life force: a term used to describe units of power

ma ha ni yom: a form of magic

Mae Phosop: the patroness of rice and rice culture

mandala: a symbol of *dharmachakra*, the Wheel of Law and endless cycle of rebirth

Mara: a demon god

maw paeng: a creator of negative power

metta: loving-kindness, benevolence, and harmony

mulberry tree (*Broussonetia papyrifera*): the inner bark is used for making Shan paper

naga: a mythical sea dragon or serpent associated with water and fertility

Nang Sulat Siwalee: protector of Buddhist scriptures

Nang Thorani: vanquisher of the demon god Mara

nar: a page of a manuscript

numerology: the mystical power of numbers

Om: short for the incantation *om mani padme hum*

paan: a mixture of betel leaf, betel nut, and slaked lime

Pali: Indo-Aryan literary and liturgical language of Theravada Buddhism written in various scripts

Pali incantation: used for healing and good luck

pap saa: a mulberry paper manuscript

pap tup: a manuscript in one sheet folded backwards and forwards to create concertina-style pleats

pap tup lik: a script

phi lo: a powerful spirit ogre, popular in Shan State

pong pheuw: a void in space that draws in suffering and unhappiness

porcupine bezoar: a stony secretion which forms in the stomach of a porcupine

positive power: supernatural power that creates good

precepts: Buddhist rules governing behaviour

Rahu: god of eclipses

saiyasart: supernaturalism considered 'not strictly Buddhist'

saya (sala): an expert in the arts of the supernatural

Shan: Tai of the Shan States

sompoy (*Accacia rugata Merr.*): a local plant used in purification rituals

Sulat Siwali: Tai form of the Hindu goddess Salasvati

sutta: sacred texts

Tai: people inhabiting Assam, the Shan States, southwest China, Laos, and Thailand who share a common heritage, of which there are many subgroups

Tai Yai (also called Shan Proper or Tai Ngio): Tai of the Shan States and western Lan Na

thao thang si: guardian spirits

thien suk lap luk: a good luck incantation

tical: 0.576 ounces (16.33 gm)

Triple Gem: the Buddha, the *sangha* (monks), and the *dhamma* (law)

ya muk: a wild plant whose sap is used as a binding material

yakka: a spirit

yantra: mystical symbolic diagrams

Folios 29–32

Bibliography

Amphay Doré. 1992. *L'école de la Forêt: un itinéraire spirituel lao*. Aurangabad, India: Kailash Books.

Becchetti, Catherine. 1991. *Le Mystere Dans Les Lettres*. Bangkok: Editions Des Cahiers de France.

Berkwitz, Stephen C.; Schober, Juliane; and Brown, Claudia, eds. 2009. *Buddhist Manuscript Cultures: Knowledge, Ritual, and Art*. New York: Routledge.

Brun, Viggo, and Schumacher, Trond. 1994. *Traditional Herbal Medicine in Northern Thailand*. Bangkok: White Lotus.

Chen L.; Wang X.; and Huang B. J. 2015. 'The Genus Hippocampus: A Review on Traditional Medicinal Uses, Chemical Constituents, and Pharmacological Properties'. *Journal of Ethnopharmacology* 162: 104–11.

Conway, Susan. 2006. *The Shan: Culture, Arts and Crafts*. Bangkok: River Books.

————. 2007a. 'Shan Buddhism and Culture'. Paper presented at the Conference on Shan Buddhism and Culture, SOAS Centre of Buddhist Studies and the Shan Cultural Association UK, December 8–9.

————. 2007b. 'Shan Expressions of Power and Protection'. In *The Secrets of Southeast Asian Textiles: Myth, Status and the Supernatural*. Bangkok: James H W Thompson Foundation.

————. 2014. *Tai Magic: Arts of the Supernatural*. Bangkok: River Books.

Davis, Richard. 1974. 'Tolerance and Intolerance of Ambiguity in Northern Thai Myth and Ritual'. *Ethnology* 13: 1–24.

Eberhardt, Nancy. 2006. *Imagining the Course of Life: Self-transformation in a Shan Buddhist Community*. Chiang Mai: Silkworm Books.

Geertz, Clifford. 1973. *The Interpretation of Cultures*. New York: Basic Books.

Ginsburg, Henry D. 1989. *Thai Manuscript Painting*. London: British Library.

Grabowsky, Volker, ed. 2022. *Manuscript Cultures and Epigraphy of the Tai World*. Chiang Mai: Silkworm Books.

Grabowsky, Volker, and Turton, Andrew, eds. 2003. *The Gold and Silver Road of Trade and Friendship: The McLeod and Richardson Diplomatic Missions to Tai States in 1837*. Chiang Mai: Silkworm Books.

Herbert, Patricia. 2002. 'Burmese Cosmological Manuscripts'. In *Burma: Art and Archaeology*, eds. Alexandra Green and T. Richard Blurton, 77–97. London: British Library.

Hsu, Jeremy, 2017. 'The Hard Truth about the Rhino Horn "Aphrodisiac" Market'. *Scientific American*, 5 April.

Iddhichiracharas, Narujohn. 1980. 'The Northern Thai Peasant Supernaturalism'. In *Buddhism in Northern Thailand*, eds. Saeng Chandrangaam and Narujohn Iddhichiracharas, 100–4. University of Chiang Mai.

Kourilsky, Gregory, and Berment, Vincent. 2005. 'Towards a Computerization of the Lao Tham System of Writing'. Paper presented at the First International Conference on Lao Studies, Dekalb, 20–22 May.

Kraisri Nimmanahaeminda. 1967. 'The Lawa Guardian Spirits of Chiangmai'. *Journal of the Siam Society* 55 (BE 2527): 185–225.

Mayoury and Pheuiphanh Ngaosrivathana. 2009. *The Enduring Sacred Landscape of the Naga*. Chiang Mai: Mekong Press.

McAlister V. 2005. 'Sacred Disease of Our Times: Failure of the Infectious Disease Model of Spongiform Encephalopathy'. Clinical and Investigative Medicine 28(3): 101–4.

McDaniel, Justin. 2009. *Gathering Leaves and Lifting Words: Histories of Buddhist Monastic Education in Laos and Thailand*. Chiang Mai: Silkworm Books.

Milne, Leslie, and Cochrane, Wilbur Willis. 1910. *Shans at Home*; reprint New York: Paragon, 1970.

Perdue, Daniel. 2002. *The Course in Buddhist Reasoning and Debate: An Asian Approach to Analytical Thinking Drawn from Indian and Tibetan Sources*. Boston MA: Shambhala Publications.

Roos, Anna Marie. 2008. '"Magic Coins" and "Magic Squares": The Discovery of Astrological Sigils in the Oldenburg Letters'. In *Notes and Records of the Royal Society* 62: 271–88.

Sai Kam Mong. 2004. *The History and Development of the Shan Scripts*. Chiang Mai: Silkworm Books.

Saimong Mangrai (Sao). 1981. *The Paedaeng Chronicle and the Jengtung State Chronicle* (translation). *Michigan Papers on South and Southeast Asia* 19. Ann Arbor: University of Michigan Center for South and Southeast Asian Studies.

San San May. 2011. 'Tattoo Art in Burmese Culture'. Southeast Asia Library Group Newsletter, 43, December.

Sheravanichkul, Arthid. 2009. 'Phu Khwan Khao Worship of Shan in Yunnan: Fertility and Buddhist Felicity'. *Contemporary Buddhism* 10(1): 159–70.

Sommai Premchit and Amphay Doré. 1992. *The Lan Na Twelve-Month Traditions: An Ethno-historic and Comparative Approach*. Chiang Mai University, Thailand, and Centre National de la Recherche Scientifique, France.

Sparkes, Stephen. 2005. *Spirits and Souls: Gender and Cosmology in an Isan Village in Northeast Thailand*. Bangkok: White Lotus.

Spiro, Melford E. 1967. *Burmese Supernaturalism: A Study in the Explanation and Reduction of Suffering*. New Jersey: Prentice-Hall.

Tambiah, Stanley Jeyaraja. 1984. *The Buddhist Saints of the Forest and the Cult of Amulets*. Cambridge: Cambridge University Press.

Tannenbaum, Nicola. 1987. 'Tattoos: Invulnerability and Power in Shan Cosmology'. *American Ethnologist* 14(4): 693–711.

Terwiel, B. J. 1994. *Monks and Magic: An Analysis of Religious Ceremonies in Central Thailand*. Bangkok: White Lotus.

Vater, Tom, and Thaewchatturat, Aroon. 2011. *Sacred Skin: Thailand's Spirit Tattoos*. Bangkok: Visionary World.

Verpoorte, Rob. 2015. 'Food and Medicine: Old Traditions, Novel Opportunities'. *Journal of Ethnobiology and Ethnomedicine* 167: 1 (editorial).

Zhu Liangwen. 1992. *The Dai, or The Tai and Their Architecture and Customs in South China*. Bangkok: DD Books.

Folios 33–36

Medicinal Index

acaia (*Acacia rugata Mer*)

agarwood (*Aquilaria*), also called eaglewood

alfalfa (*Medicago sativa*)

ambergris, secretion from the intestine of a sperm whale (*Physeter catodon*)

anise (*Illicium verum*)

aromatic ginger (*Kaempferia galangal*)

asafoetida (*Ferula apiaceae*), known as 'devil's dung'

bael fruit (*Aegle marmelos*), also called stone fruit

bastard sandalwood (*Mansonia gagei*)

bayan fig (*Ficus benghalensis*)

beehive ginger (*Zingiber spectabile*)

bitter bottle gourd (*Lagenaria siceraria*)

bitter cucumber (*Colocynth*)

bitter gourd (*Momordica charantia*)

bitter oleander (*Holarrhena pubescens*)

black bat lily (*Tacca chantrieri*)

black bean root (*Sophora exigua* Craib.)

black cardamom (*Amomum subulatum*)

black leadwort (*Plumbago auriculata*)

black myrobalan (*Terminalia chebula*)

black nightshade (*Solanum nigrum*)

black sacred garlic pear (*Crateva religiosa*)

black turmeric (*Curcuma caesia*)

blackberry lily (*Belamcanda chinensis*)

blackboard tree (*Alstonia scholaris*)

blue fountain bush (*Clerodendrum serratum*)

blue lotus (*Nymphaea nouchali*)

borax, sodium borate

bowing lady flower (*Clerodendron siphonanthus*)

brown love grass (*Eragrostiella*)

bush weed (*Flueggea virosa*)

candy lily (*Belamcanda chinensis*)

castor bean (*Ricinus communis*)

Ceylon oak (*Schleichera oleosa*)

chamber bitter (*Phyllanthus urinaria*)

chaulmoongra (*Hydrocarpus wightianus*)

cherimoya (*Annona cherimola*)

Chinese finger ginger (*Boesenbergia rotunda*)

Chinese laurel (*Antidesma bunius*)

Christmas bush (*Chromolaena odorata*), also called Siam weed

cinammon tree (*Cinnamomum verum*)

climbing wattle (*Senegalia pennata*)

common bushweed (*Flueggea virosa*)

croton (*Croton oblongifolius* Roxb.)

devil's horsewhip (*Achyranthes aspera*)

devil's ivy (*Epipremnum aureum*), also called money plant

devil's tree (*Alstonia scholaris*)

devil's trumpet (*Datura stramonium*)

dodder (*Cuscuta*)

dog bush (*Blumea balsamifera*)

drooping fig (*Ficus semicordata*)

drumstick tree (*Moringa tree*)

dwarf Indian olive (*Elaeocarpus robustus*)

dwarf umbrella plant (*Schefflera arboricol*)

elephant ear fig tree (*Ficus auriculata*), also called night-scented lily

elephant ear plant (*Alocasia odora*)

elephant grass (*Arundo donax*)

entada bean (*Entada phaseoloides*)

false daisy (*Eclipta alba*)

fever nut (*Caesaplinia bonduc (L.) Roxb.*)

ficus (*Ficus benjamina*), also called weeping fig

fig (*Ficus carica*)

fishtail palm (*Caryota mitis*)

flaming lily (*Gloriosa superba*)

fragrant anneslea (*Anneslea fragarans*)

fragrant bay (*Machilus odoratissima*)

freshwater mangrove (*Carallia brachiate*)

giant bamboo (*Dendrocalamus giganteus*)

giant fern tree (*Angiopteris avecta*)

ginger (*Hitchenia glauca*)

golden shower tree (*Cassia fistula*)

golden thread vine (*Cuscuta pacifica*)

green milkweed climber (*Dregea volubilis*)

grey nicker (*Caesalpinia crista*)

guduchi (*Tinospora cordifolia*), also called heart-leaved moonseed

heart-leaved moonseed (*Tinospora cordifolia*)

heliotrope (*Heliotropiaceae*)

Himalayan gentian (*Gentian kurroo*)

holy basil (*Ocimum tenuiflorum*)

Indian bay seed (*Cinnamomum tamala*)
Indian birthwort (*Aristolochia tagala*)
Indian ginseng (*Withania somnifera*), also called winter cherry
Indian gooseberry (*Phyllanthus emblica*)
Indian ipecac (*Tylophora indica*)
Indian ivy rue (*Zanthoxylum rhetsa*)
Indian jujube (*Ziziphus Mauritania*)
Indian lotus (*Nelumbo nucifera*), also called sacred water lily
Indian sarsaparilla (*Hemidesmus indicus*)
Indian snake root (*Rauwolfia serpentina*)
Indian trumpet tree (*Oroxylum indicum*)
Indian valerian (*Valeriana wallichii*)
Indian wild liquorice (*Abrus precatorius*)
Indian wild pepper (*Vitex trifolia*)

Jamaican wild liquorice (*Abrus precatorius linn.*)
Japanese climbing fern (*Lygodium japonicum*)
Japanese yam (*Dioscorea japonica*)
Java bean (*Senna obtusifolia*)

lemon basil (*Ocimum basillicum*)
lemon vine (*Pereskia aculeata*)
liquorice (*Glycyrrhiza glabra*)
long pepper (*Piper longum*)

Malabar nut (*Justicia adhatoda*)
mat daisy (*Anacyclus pyrethrum*)
milk hedge (*Euphorbia nivulia*)
millettia (*Millettia racemosa* Roxb.)

mistletoe (*Viscum cruciatum*)

money plant (*Epipremnum aureum*)

monkey jack (*Artocarpus lacucha*), also called monkey fruit

monkey pod tree (*Samanea saman*), also called rain tree

moonseed (*Menispermu*)

mugwort (*Artemisia absinthium*)

needle wood tree (*Schima wallichii*)

nicker seed (*Caesalpinia crista*)

night-scented lily (*Alocasia odora*), also called elephant ear plant

nutgall black seed (*Rhus Javanica*)

orchid tree (*Bauhinia purpurea*)

paper mulberry (*Broussonetia papyrifera*)

physic nut (*Jatrophe cursas L.*)

pipe vine (*Aristolochia macrophylla*)

pomegranate (*Punica granatum*)

potato tree (*Solanum erianthum*)

purging croton (*Croton tiglium*)

pygmy water lily (*Nymphaea tetragona*)

quince seed (*Cydonia oblong*)

rain tree (*Samanea saman*)

red castor bean (*Ricinus communis*)

red water lily (*Nymphaea rubra*)

rex begonia vine (*Cissus javana*)

ridge gourd (*Luffa acutangula*)

Ridley's staghorn fern (*Platycerium ridleyi*)

rosy leadwort (*Plumbago indica*)

rosary pea (*Abrus precatorius*), also called jequirity bean

sacred garlic pear (*Crateva religiosa*)
sacred water lily (*Nelumbo nucifera*)
sal ammoniac, ammonium chloride
shikakai (*Senegalia rugata* Lam.)
Siamese cassia buds (*Senna siamea*)
silk tree (*Albizia chinansis*)
snowflake tree (*Trevesia palmata*)
snuffbox sea bean (*Entada rheedii*)
soap pods (*Senegalia rugata*)
St. Thomas lid pod (*Perculina turpethum*)
stink vine (*Paederia foetida)*
stone apple (*Aegle marmelos*)
stone ginger (*Rrhynchanthus longiflorus*)
strychnine (*Strychnos nux-vomica*)
sweet basil (*Ocimum basilicum*)
sweet flag (*Acorus calamus*)
sweet indrajao (*Wrightia tinctoria*)
sweet wood (*Glycyrrhiza glabra*)

tagara (Indian valerian)
tailed pepper (*Piper tubeba*)
tea (*Camellia sinensis*)
thorn apple (*Datura stramonium*)
toothbrush tree (*Salvadora persica*)
tube flower (*Clerodendron siphonanthus*)
turpeth (*Operculina turpethum*)

velvet nightshade (*Solanum erianthum*)

water pepper (*Persicaria hydropiper*)

white dammar tree (*Vateria indica*)

white leadwort (*Plumbago zeylanica*)

white turmeric root (*Curcuma zedoaria*)

white water lily (*Nymphaea alba*)

white water lily (small) (*Nymphaea tetragona georgi*)

white willow tree (*Salix alba*)

wild asparagus (*Asparagus prostrates*)

wild croton (*Baliospermum montanum*)

wild ginger (*Zingiber cassumunar* Roxb.)

wild pepper (*Vitex trifolia*)

willow-leaved justicia (*Justicia gendarussa*), also called shrimp plant

winter cherry (*Withania somnifera*)

wireweed (*Polygonella basiramia*)

woolly dyeing rosebay (*Wrightia orborea*)

yellow damson (*Chrysophyllum oliviforme*)

yellow jade orchid tree (*Magnolia champaca*)

zebrawood (*Pistacia integerrima*)

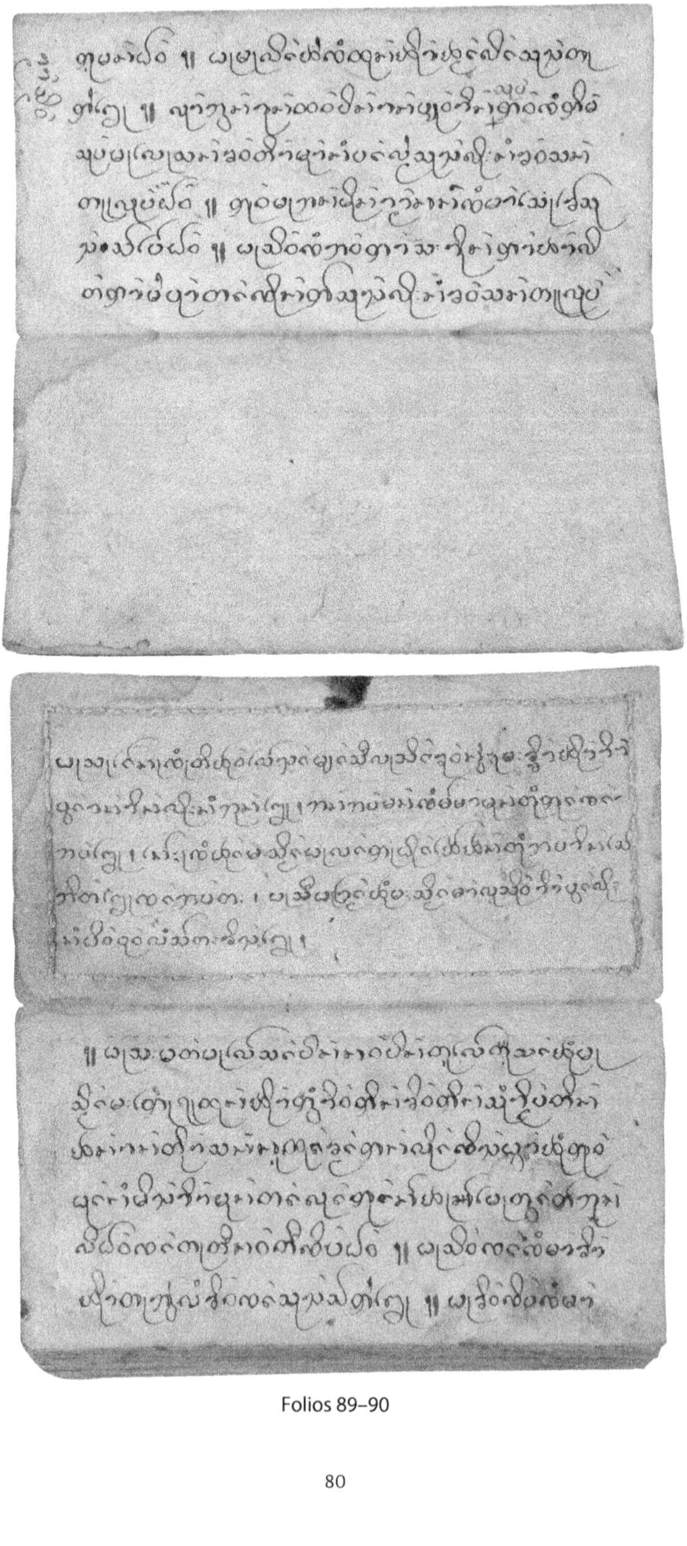

Folios 89–90

Acknowledgments

I would like to express my gratitude to Phra Dhammsami, Rector of Shan State Buddhist University, Shan State, Myanmar. Also to Phra Viccita, Abbot of Shan State Buddhist University, who supported translation of this text from an ancient Shan script into modern Shan, and to Zaray Saw (Sai Seng), student of Shan manuscripts, who gave advice. Thanks also go to my Shan MA students, both monks and lay members of the community, who provided information on Shan village rituals.

In Keng Tung, Shan State, thanks go to *saya* Lung Saw Jing and *saya* Maha Kaew. I am grateful to Phra Sai Khemacari from Wat Chieng Yin, Keng Tung; Phraku Wasan from Wat Ho Khong, Keng Tung; librarian Phra Sitilong; and the monks of Wat In, Keng Tung, who gave generously of their time. I would also like to thank Tun Yee for acting as a go-between with *saya* Long Te Za, who is Shan, and *saya* Long Noi Na, who is Tai Yuan. They provided the list of illnesses, healing incantations, and magic spells used in the text.

Details of Shan belief systems were explained to me by Phrakru Wimonsilapakij of Mahachulalongkornrajavidyalaya University, Chiang Rai; Kam Indra and Phra Payongsak at Wat Pa Daed, Chiang Mai; and Phra Jeruwana Yeenoon and Phra Supachai Chayasupho at Wat Suan Dork, Chiang Mai. I was invited to observe healing rituals administered by Phra Warinda and the monks of Wat Tiyasathan, Mae Daeng. Thanks also go to the herbalist and spirit medium Nang Lord. In Mae Hong Son, I am grateful to Khun Yai Yotmanee, Khun Gaysorn, Khun Kan-na (Sua Yen)

Rubnamtham, Lung Ae Piya Wong, Acharn Baan Langkhu, and Khun Long Tan Kyo.

Thanks go to Dr Fiona Kerlogue, who first alerted me to the presence of this manuscript in the collections of the Horniman Museum and Gardens, London. I would also like to thank the Asia Department at the Library of Congress, Washington DC. The Rockefeller Foundation, New York, provided funding for fieldwork and for publication of this book. I am grateful to Melissa Leach, Director of the Institute of Development Studies, University of Sussex, and to Mariz Tadros, Fellow at the Institute of Development Studies, University of Sussex.

Finally, I wish to thank my publisher Trasvin Jittidecharak of Silkworm Books, Chiang Mai, and Nang Hseng Noung who worked so hard on the Shan to English translation.

Printed in the USA
CPSIA information can be obtained
at www.ICGtesting.com
CBHW042057010424
6229CB00001B/1